Cardiovascular MRI

CONTEMPORARY CARDIOLOGY

CHRISTOPHER P. CANNON, MD
SERIES EDITOR

ANNEMARIE M. ARMANI, MD
EXECUTIVE EDITOR

Cardiovascular MRI: *150 Multiple-Choice Questions and Answers, by Peter G. Danias, MD, PHD, 2008*

Pulmonary Hypertension, edited by *Nicholas S. Hill, and Harrison W. Farber, MD, 2008*

Nuclear Cardiology: *The Basics: How to Set Up and Maintain a Laboratory, Second Edition,* ***by*** *Frans Wackers, MD, PHD, Barry L. Zaret, MD, PHD, and Wendy Bruni, CNMT, 2008*

Rapid ECG Interpretation, Third Edition, by *M. Gabriel Khan, MD, FRCP, 2008*

Therapeutic Lipidology, edited by *Michael H. Davidson, MD, Kevin C. Maki, PHD, and Peter P. Toth, MD, PHD, 2007*

Essentials of Restenosis: *For the Interventional Cardiologist,* ***edited by*** *Henricus J. Duckers, PHD, MD, Patrick W. Serruys, MD, and Elizabeth G. Nabel, MD, 2007*

Cardiac Drug Therapy, *Seventh Edition,* ***by*** *M. Gabriel Khan, MD, FRCP, 2007*

Cardiovascular Magnetic Resonance Imaging, edited by *Raymond Y. Kwong, MD, 2007*

Essential Echocardiography: *A Practical Handbook With DVD,* ***edited by*** *Scott D. Solomon, MD, 2007*

Cardiac Rehabilitation, edited by *William Kraus, MD, and Steven Keteyian, MD*

Management of Acute Pulmonary Embolism, edited by *Stavros Konstantinides, MD, 2007*

Stem Cells and Myocardial Regeneration, edited by *Marc S. Penn, MD, PHD, 2007*

Handbook of Complex Percutaneous Carotid Intervention, edited by *Jacqueline Saw, MD, Jose Exaire, MD, David S. Lee, MD, Sanjay Yadav, MD, 2007*

Preventive Cardiology: *Insights Into the Prevention and Treatment of Cardiovascular Disease, Second Edition,* ***edited by*** *JoAnne Micale Foody, MD, 2007*

The Art and Science of Cardiac Physical Examination: *With Heart Sounds and Pulse Wave Forms on CD,* ***by*** *Narasimhan Ranganathan, MD, Vahe Sivaciyan, MD, and Franklin B. Saksena, MD, 2006*

Cardiovascular Biomarkers: *Pathophysiology and Disease Management,* ***edited by*** *David A. Morrow, MD, 2006*

Cardiovascular Disease in the Elderly, edited by *Gary Gerstenblith, MD, 2005*

Platelet Function: *Assessment, Diagnosis, and Treatment,* ***edited by*** *Martin Quinn, MB BCH BAO, PHD, and Desmond Fitzgerald, MD, FRCPI, FESC, APP, 2005*

Diabetes and Cardiovascular Disease, *Second Edition,* ***edited by*** *Michael T. Johnstone, MD, CM, FRCP(C), and Aristidis Veves, MD, DSC, 2005*

Angiogenesis and Direct Myocardial Revascularization, edited by *Roger J. Laham, MD, and Donald S. Baim, MD, 2005*

Interventional Cardiology: *Percutaneous Noncoronary Intervention,* ***edited by*** *Howard C. Herrmann, MD, 2005*

Principles of Molecular Cardiology, edited by *Marschall S. Runge, MD, and Cam Patterson, MD, 2005*

Heart Disease Diagnosis and Therapy: *A Practical Approach, Second Edition,* ***by*** *M. Gabriel Khan, MD, FRCP(LONDON), FRCP(C), FACP, FACC, 2005*

Cardiovascular Genomics: *Gene Mining for Pharmacogenomics and Gene Therapy,* ***edited by*** *Mohan K. Raizada, PHD, Julian F. R. Paton, PHD, Michael J. Katovich, PHD, and Sergey Kasparov, MD, PHD, 2005*

Surgical Management of Congestive Heart Failure, edited by *James C. Fang, MD and Gregory S. Couper, MD, 2005*

Cardiopulmonary Resuscitation, edited by *Joseph P. Ornato, MD, FACP, FACC, FACEP and Mary Ann Peberdy, MD, FACC, 2005*

CT of the Heart: *Principles and Applications,* ***edited by*** *U. Joseph Schoepf, MD, 2005*

Coronary Disease in Women: *Evidence-Based Diagnosis and Treatment,* ***edited by*** *Leslee J. Shaw, PHD and Rita F. Redberg, MD, FACC, 2004*

Cardiac Transplantation: *The Columbia University Medical Center/New York-Presbyterian Hospital Manual,* ***edited by*** *Niloo M. Edwards, MD, Jonathan M. Chen, MD, and Pamela A. Mazzeo, 2004*

Heart Disease and Erectile Dysfunction, edited by *Robert A. Kloner, MD, PHD, 2004*

Complementary and Alternative Cardiovascular Medicine, edited by *Richard A. Stein, MD and Mehmet C. Oz, MD, 2004*

Nuclear Cardiology, The Basics: *How to Set Up and Maintain a Laboratory,* ***by*** *Frans J. Th. Wackers, MD, PHD, Wendy Bruni, BS, CNMT, and Barry L. Zaret, MD, 2004*

Minimally Invasive Cardiac Surgery, Second Edition, edited by *Daniel J. Goldstein, MD, and Mehmet C. Oz, MD 2004*

Cardiovascular Health Care Economics, edited by *William S. Weintraub, MD, 2003*

Platelet Glycoprotein IIb/IIIa Inhibitors in Cardiovascular Disease, *Second Edition,* ***edited by*** *A. Michael Lincoff, MD, 2003*

Heart Failure: *A Clinician's Guide to Ambulatory Diagnosis and Treatment,* ***edited by*** *Mariell L. Jessup, MD and Evan Loh, MD, 2003*

Management of Acute Coronary Syndromes, *Second Edition,* ***edited by*** *Christopher P. Cannon, MD 2003*

Aging, Heart Disease, and Its Management: *Facts and Controversies,* ***edited by*** *Niloo M. Edwards, MD, Mathew S. Maurer, MD, and Rachel B. Wellner, MPH, 2003*

Peripheral Arterial Disease: *Diagnosis and Treatment,* ***edited by*** *Jay D. Coffman, MD and Robert T. Eberhardt, MD, 2003*

Cardiac Repolarization: *Bridging Basic and Clinical Science,* ***edited by*** *Ihor Gussak, MD, PHD, Charles Antzelevitch, PHD, Step*[redacted] *Shen, MD, and Preben* [redacted]

Cardiovascular MRI

150 Multiple Choice Questions and Answers

Peter G. Danias, MD, PHD

Cardiac MR Center, Hygeia Hospital, Athens, Greece
Tufts University School of Medicine, Boston, MA

Foreword by Warren J. Manning, MD

Humana Press

Peter G. Danias, MD, PhD
Adjunct Associate Professor of Medicine
Tufts University School of Medicine
Boston, MA
Cardiac MR Center
Hygeia Hospital
Maroussi, Athens, Greece
peter.danias@tufts.edu
pdanias@hygeia.gr

ISBN: 978-1-934115-59-6 e-ISBN: 978-1-59745-511-4

Library of Congress Control Number: 2007941653

Printed on acid-free paper

9 8 7 6 5 4 3 2 1

springer.com

To my parents, brother, and teachers who made me who I am and helped me get this far.

To my beloved wife Mary, our lovely daughter Katerina, and our newborn son, who are the light in my life and keep me going.

Foreword

It has now been 20 years since I was a cardiology fellow and viewed my first cardiovascular magnetic resonance (CMR) image. This seminal event in my career occurred during an otherwise unremarkable Wednesday morning cardiac catheterization conference. Dr. Sven Paulin, Chief of Radiology at the former Beth Israel Hospital, Boston, showed us a cine ECG-triggered gradient-echo CMR study in a patient with severe aortic regurgitation. Although crude by today's standards, this cine image with obvious valvular dysfunction "took my breath away" and led me on my noninvasive imaging career.

Since then, CMR has evolved from a somewhat laborious research tool with "great potential" to a widely used and multifaceted clinical tool with a multitude of rapid imaging sequences used by clinicians around the globe to advance our understanding of cardiovascular disease and the care of our patients. We have witnessed the development of CMR-focused societies composed of clinicians and scientists, such as the Society for Cardiovascular Magnetic Resonance and European Cardiac MR Working Group, as well as the publication of guidelines by the American College of Cardiology, European Society of Cardiology, and Society for Cardiovascular Magnetic Resonance for the clinical use of CMR. With this growth has come the important issue of CMR training for our cardiovascular fellows and radiology residents/fellows as well as the education and training of the much larger number of cardiovascular imaging practitioners who have completed their formal training.

The versatility of CMR for assessment of cardiac anatomy, function, viability, perfusion, blood flow, ischemia, and vasculature has always been both its great strength and great weakness. Strength for the ability of CMR to provide a comprehensive assessment of cardiovascular physiology and pathology; weakness because of the inherent complexity of CMR—tissues may be black, gray, or white depending on the sequence and underlying pathology and the use of an exogenous contrast agent. "It is so complex" are the words often expressed by those new to the field. Indeed, guidelines for fellowship training and postgraduate training for the clinical practice of CMR include substantial didactic efforts to fully appreciate and harness the power of CMR.

Although formal CMR textbooks are widely available, Dr. Danias has provided us with a unique, thematically organized, multiple choice question and answer format text to learn and to test our knowledge of CMR. CMR practitioners at all levels will find this text useful because of its clarity in presentation and wide breadth of coverage, with the added value of references for those who wish to pursue more in-depth discussions.

The question is no longer "when" will CMR have a clinical role, but rather "which patient" and using what sequence/application. Dr. Danias has provided us with a valuable learning tool that will benefit both the new and the seasoned CMR practitioner. As the field continues to advance, I look forward to the next 150 questions!

Warren J. Manning, MD
Professor of Medicine and Radiology
Harvard Medical School
Section Chief of Non-invasive
Cardiac Imaging
Beth Israel Deaconess Medical Center
Boston, MA, USA

Preface

The recent rapid growth of cardiovascular magnetic resonance imaging (CMR) has reflected the trend of modern Medicine towards increasing development and utilization of noninvasive diagnostic approaches. CMR is particularly appealing because it can assess every aspect of cardiovascular anatomy, physiology, and pathology with exquisite accuracy, precision, and most importantly, with minimal associated biologic risks.

This textbook aims to provide a comprehensive educational tool for physicians who start getting involved with CMR and for the cardiology and radiology trainees who study for Board certification. The book includes 150 multiple choice questions and answers with concise explanation on each question and pertinent up-to-date bibliography.

The textbook includes chapters on physics and safety, general CMR, valvular heart disease, diseases of the myocardium and pericardium, ischemic heart disease, congenital heart disease, and diseases of the great vessels. The questions, many of which are based on clinical cases, are constructed so as to bring up teaching points. Each of the chapters is a separate entity, although the first two chapters provide the necessary background knowledge to build on for the subsequent ones.

All 135 images included in this textbook were obtained from patient studies performed at the CMR Center of Hygeia Hospital, a tertiary referral center in Athens, Greece, and a Harvard Medical International Affiliate. Sincere thanks to all our patients and to all the staff of the CT and MRI department for their support of this effort. And last but not least, many thanks to all my teachers and colleagues at the Beth Israel Deaconess Medical Center in Boston who helped me start my career in CMR.

Peter G. Danias, MD, PHD

Contents

1

Physics and Safety

Peter G. Danias, *Cardiovascular MRI: 150 Multiple-Choice Questions and Answers*

1. The magnetic field strength (1.5 T) routinely used for cardiovascular magnetic resonance imaging (CMR) is:

A. Roughly equal to the earth's magnetic field
B. One hundred times stronger than the earth's magnetic field
C. One thousand times stronger than the earth's magnetic field
D. Thirty thousand times stronger than the earth's magnetic field
E. One hundred and twenty thousand times stronger than the earth's magnetic field

Correct answer is D.

The strength of a magnetic field may be measured in tesla (T) or gauss. One tesla is equal to 10,000 gauss. The earth's magnetic field at the earth's surface varies between 0.3 and 0.6 gauss. Most clinical CMR scanners use a magnetic field of 1.5 T, or 15,000 gauss, i.e., approximately 30,000 times stronger than the earth's magnetic field. [1, 2]

2. For magnetic resonance imaging (MRI), the signal that is used to create the image is emitted from:

A. The carbon-12 nuclei (C^{12})
B. The oxygen-16 nuclei (O^{16})
C. The nitrogen-14 nuclei (N^{14})
D. The hydrogen nuclei (H^{1})
E. The carbon-12 electron cloud

Correct answer is D.

When nuclei are placed inside a magnetic field, they are aligned parallel or antiparallel to the field orientation and precess, if they have an odd number of protons [2]. For routine clinical MRI, the signal is derived from the precession of the hydrogen nuclei. There are mainly two advantages in using hydrogen for this purpose: first, it is greatly abundant, because it is part of the water molecule. Second, its gyromagnetic ratio (42.6×10^6 Hz/T) provides for an optimal resonant frequency (63.8 MHz) at 1.5 T. Other nuclei used for imaging (mostly with high-field systems) include sodium-23 (Na^{23}) and fluoride-19 (F^{19}) [2].

3. In a 1.5-T scanner, the resonance frequency for the hydrogen protons is:

A. 63 Hz
B. 63 kHz
C. 63 MHz
D. 63 GHz
E. Depends on the tissue to be imaged

Correct answer is C.

The resonance frequency of the nuclei inside a magnetic field is derived by the Larmor equation: $\omega = \gamma \times B_o$, where ω is the resonance frequency, γ is the gyromagnetic ratio, and B_0 is the magnetic field strength. The gyromagnetic ratio for hydrogen is 42.58×10^6 Hz/T [3], thus, for a field strength of 1.5 T, the hydrogen resonance frequency is $(1.5 \times 42.58 \times 10^6) = 63.87$ MHz. It is important to remember that the radiofrequency (RF) pulses used for routine clinical MRI are in the FM range.

4. When material is placed inside a strong magnetic field, the hydrogen nuclei:

A. Align all their spins parallel to the direction of the main magnetic field
B. Align their spins either parallel or opposite to the direction of the main magnetic field
C. Start interacting with each other, resulting in T1 relaxation
D. Loose energy, resulting in T2 decay
E. Stop precessing

Correct answer is B.

When material is placed inside a strong magnetic field, the hydrogen nuclei tend to align their spins either parallel or opposite to the direction of the main magnetic field. The parallel orientation is slightly favored, because it is a lower energy state [4, 5]. For every one million protons counter aligned to the magnetic field, there will be one million and ten spins aligned in the direction of the field [2]. T1 relaxation and T2 decay occur only after the material is stimulated with a RF resonant pulse that will deliver energy to the tissue.

5. An object constructed from ferromagnetic material placed inside a static magnetic field will have:

A. Higher field strength inside the object than around it
B. The same field strength inside and outside the object
C. Lower field strength inside the object than around it
D. Minimal (if any) magnetic susceptibility
E. Electric current generated inside the object

Correct answer is A.

Ferromagnetic materials (such as iron, nickel, or cobalt) have a large positive magnetic susceptibility, i.e., when placed in a magnetic field, the field strength is much stronger inside the material than outside. Paramagnetic material (such as gadolinium, oxygen, and magnesium) have a weak positive susceptibility (<1/1,000 compared with ferromagnetic materials). Diamagnetic materials (such as copper, nitrogen, water, and most biologic tissues) have small negative magnetic susceptibility, i.e., when placed inside a magnetic field, the field strength is slightly lower inside the material than outside [6]. Electric current is not generated inside an object unless the object is moving inside the magnetic field (or the field changes over time).

6. T1 relaxation time is the time that it takes for the longitudinal magnetization of excited tissues to return to what percent of the original value?

A. 50%
B. 63%
C. 86%
D. 95%
E. 100%

Correct answer is B.

T1 relaxation is characterized by the return of the net magnetization to its basic state of maximum length in the direction of the main magnetic field. The rate of the return of the longitudinal magnetization depends on the interaction of the spins with the surrounding nuclei (spin-lattice relaxation) and is an exponential process. T1 is the constant that describes this exponential process. Thus, in time = T1, 63% of the magnetization will have recovered; in time 2 × T1, 86%; in time 3 × T1, 95%, etc. [2]

7. Which of the following statements regarding T2 is correct?

A. T2 relaxation results from exchange of energy between adjacent spins and with the surrounding lattice
B. T2 relaxation occurs both in the transverse and longitudinal orientations
C. In biologic tissues, T2 is higher than T1
D. In pure water, T1 and T2 are approximately equal
E. In time equal to T2, 50% of the transverse magnetization will be lost

Correct answer is D.

T2 or transverse relaxation occurs when adjacent spins in the high- and low-energy state exchange energy, but without loss of energy to the surrounding lattice. In pure water, T1 and T2 are similar (2–3 s), but, in biologic tissues, T2 is considerably lower than T1 (e.g., T2 for fat is 84 ms and for muscle is 47 ms, whereas T1 at 1.0 T for fat is 240 ms and for muscle is 730 ms). The T2 decay is an exponential curve. Thus, in time equal to T2, 63% of the transverse magnetization will be lost [2].

8. Which of the following statements is correct regarding MRI of biologic tissues?

A. T1 (longitudinal, spin-lattice relaxation) is shorter than T2 (transverse, spin-spin relaxation)
B. Fluids have long T1 and T2 values
C. Fluids and fat both have long T1 values
D. Fluids and fat both have short T1 values
E. T1 is equal to T2 for most tissues

Correct answer is B.

Biologic tissues have characteristic T1 and T2 values. T1 is longer than T2. Fluids have long T1 and T2 values (mnemonic: long drinks). Fat tissue has short T1 and T2 values (mnemonic: fast food) [2, 4, 7, 8].

9. Which of the following statements is correct?

A. The T1 value for water is approximately 100 ms
B. The T1 values for biologic tissues remain essentially unchanged or slightly decrease with increasing magnetic field strength
C. The T2 values for biologic tissues increase with increasing magnetic field strength
D. The T2 values for biologic tissues remain essentially unchanged or slightly decrease with increasing magnetic field strength
E. The T2 value for normal myocardium is approximately 1,000 ms

Correct answer is D.

Tables 1.1 and 1.2 provide the in vivo calculated T1 and T2 values for biologic tissues at the commonly used magnetic field strengths (1.5 T and 3 T) [8]. T1 values increase with increasing magnetic field strength [7, 8], whereas T2 values are essentially unchanged [7] or slightly decrease [8].

Table 1.1 T1 constants

	1.5T (ms)	3.0T (ms)	% increase	*P* value
Muscle	1,130 ± 91.7	1,420 ± 38.1	20.4	0.002
Cartilage	1,060 ± 155	1,240 ± 107	14.5	0.04
Synovial fluid	2,850 ± 279	3,620 ± 320	21.2	0.01
Subcutaneous fat	288 ± 8.42	371 ± 7.94	22.3	0.0001
Marrow fat	288 ± 5.27	365 ± 9.0	21.1	0.0001

Data from [8].

Table 1.2 T2 constants

	1.5T (ms)	3.0T (ms)	% decrease	*P* value
Muscle	35.3 ± 3.85	31.7 ± 1.90	10.1	0.02
Cartilage	42.1 ± 7.05	36.9 ± 3.81	12.3	0.007
Synovial fluid	1,210 ± 140	767 ± 48.8	36.6	0.0002
Subcutaneous fat	165 ± 5.50	133 ± 4.43	19.3	0.0001
Marrow fat	165 ± 4.96	133 ± 6.14	19.3	0.0001

Data from [8].

10. In a typical T1-weighted spin-echo sequence:

A. Fat and fluids both have high signal (appear bright)
B. Fat and fluids both have low signal (appear dark)
C. Fat has high signal (appears bright) and fluids have low signal (appear dark)
D. Fat has low signal (appears dark) and fluids have high signal (appear bright)
E. Fat has intermediate signal (appears grey) and fluids have high signal (appear bright)

Correct answer is C.

Fat is bright in both T1- and T2-weighted sequences. In T1-weighted spin-echo sequences, static (or slow-flowing) fluids are dark [2, 4, 5]. Fast-flowing fluids are also dark, because by the time the readout is performed, the excited spins have moved outside the image plane [4].

11. In a typical T2-weighted spin-echo sequence:

A. Fat has low signal (appears dark)
B. Stationary/stagnant fluids have high signal (appear bright)
C. Stationary/stagnant fluids have low signal (appear dark)
D. Fat has high signal (appears bright) and stationary/stagnant fluids have low signal (appear dark)
E. Fat has intermediate signal (appears grey) and stationary/stagnant fluids have low signal (appear dark)

Correct answer is B.

Fat is bright in both T1- and T2-weighted sequences. In T2-weighted spin-echo sequences, static (or slow-flowing) fluids are bright [2, 4, 5]. This is a quick way to determine whether a sequence has mostly T2 weighting. Similar to T1-weighted sequences, in a typical T2-weighted spin-echo sequence, fast-flowing fluids are dark, because by the time the readout is performed, the excited spins have moved outside the image plane [4].

12. What happens with the electromagnetic radiation absorption when the strength of the magnetic field doubles?

A. Increases
B. Decreases
C. Remains the same
D. Largely depends on the receiver coil
E. Largely depends on the tissue to be imaged

Correct answer is A.

As the magnetic field strength increases, the resonant frequency increases as dictated by the Larmor equation ($\omega = \gamma \times B_0$, where ω is the resonance frequency, γ is the gyromagnetic ratio, and B_0 is the field strength). Accordingly, the electromagnetic radiation absorption increases. This is a major limitation of high-field imaging, where the absorbed radiation (non-ionizing) becomes an impediment for certain imaging sequences or enhancements [6].

13. Which of the following statements is correct regarding MRI generation?

A. Raw data are directly translated into pixel intensity via back projection
B. Raw data are converted to image data via Fourier transformation
C. K-space, the mathematical (virtual) space containing the image information is filled by the step-by-step frequency encoding
D. The number of phase encoding steps used for image generation depends on the size of the field-of-view
E. K-space, the mathematical (virtual) space containing the image information, is strictly a two-dimensional space; additional dimensions require L, M, N space, etc.

Correct answer is B.

K-space is a mathematical (virtual) space containing the image information. K-space can have multiple dimensions. For example, for three-dimensional sequences, k-space is also three-dimensional; for spectroscopy, k-space is four-dimensional; etc. The data in a two-dimensional k-space include frequency and phase information. The frequency and phase information are translated into image data via Fourier transformation. Phase-encoding is typically performed in a step-like fashion. For Cartesian k-space, the steps are individual lines; for spiral k-space, the steps are spirals; for radial k-space, the steps are radii; etc. The number of phase-encoding steps determines the spatial resolution and, thus, the time to acquire the image data, but does not depend on the field-of-view. Back projection is an image reconstruction technique frequently used in computed tomography (CT) scanning and nuclear imaging, but not in MRI.

14. In a CMR scan, the field-of-view is 300 × 300 mm and the matrix used for image reconstruction is 512 × 256. What is the spatial resolution for this image?

A. $2 \times 2\,mm^2$
B. $0.6 \times 1.2\,mm^2$
C. $1.7 \times 0.9\,mm^2$
D. $1 \times 1\,mm^2$
E. $1.2 \times 1.2\,mm^2$

Correct answer is B.

In this image, the 300 × 300 mm (field-of-view) is “fitted” inside the matrix 512 × 256. Accordingly, the spatial resolution is (300/512) mm × (300/256) mm = 0.6 × 1.2 mm^2.

15. A patient undergoing CMR has a heart rate of 60 beats per minute. To assess ventricular function, the operator decides to acquire a cine image with 25 phases per cardiac cycle. What is the temporal resolution for this study?

A. 25 ms
B. 40 ms
C. 50 ms
D. 60 ms
E. 80 ms

Correct answer is B.

The duration of the cardiac (RR) cycle for this patient is 1,000 ms. This time period is divided into the 25 phases that the operator elected to acquire. Thus, each phase spans 40 ms and this is the temporal resolution of this cine study. It has been shown that at least 11 phases need to be acquired to have accurate measurements of left ventricular volumes, ejection fraction, and mass [9].

16. Signal-to-noise ratio (SNR) is an important consideration in CMR. Which of the following statements is correct regarding SNR?

A. For a constant field-of-view, increasing the reconstruction matrix will increase the SNR
B. High SNR allows the differentiation of two adjacent tissues with similar magnetic properties
C. SNR is adversely affected by motion
D. Obtaining multiple averages will increase the SNR by a factor equal to the number of averages obtained
E. SNR depends on the phase encoding steps of the imaging sequence

Correct answer is E.

SNR is usually defined as the difference in signal intensity at a region of interest inside the tissue of interest minus the signal intensity outside the body (in the air), divided by the standard deviation of the signal from the background noise [2]. For a constant-sized voxel, an increase in phase-encoding steps also improves the SNR by the square root of the number of phase-encoding steps. In theory, SNR is also proportional to the volume of the voxel and to the square root of the number or averages obtained. Therefore, SNR decreases if the matrix size increases (for a fixed field-of-view). It is high contrast-to-noise ratio (CNR) and not SNR that will allow differentiation of two tissues with similar magnetic properties. SNR is not affected by motion, although image quality may be significantly degraded.

17. According to theory, what happens to the SNR when the magnetic field increases by a factor of 2?

A. Remains constant
B. Increases by a factor of 2
C. Increases by a factor of 3
D. Increases by a factor of 4
E. Decreases by a factor of 2

Correct answer is B.

The signal is proportional to the square of the magnetic field strength, and the noise is proportional to the field strength [2]. Thus, when the field strength doubles, the SNR also doubles.

18. In high magnetic fields, the magnetohydrodynamic effect affects primarily which part of the surface ECG?

A. The P complex
B. The PQ interval
C. The QRS complex
D. The ST interval
E. The UP interval

Correct answer is D.

When electrically charged particles move inside a magnetic field, electricity is produced and the induced current is proportional to the velocity of the moving particles and to the field strength. In the bloodstream, there are many electrically charged particles (ions, macromolecules, etc.). The velocity of the blood flow is greatest during ventricular ejection, which occurs during the ST segment of the ECG. Accordingly, the electric current that is produced "contaminates" the surface ECG and this affects predominantly the ST segment [10]. This is the reason why the ECG cannot be used inside the magnet to assess for ischemia, but only for rhythm detection.

19. The basic difference between spin-echo and gradient-echo sequences is:

A. Spin-echo sequences are faster than gradient-echo sequences
B. Spin-echo sequences have T1- or T2-weighting, whereas gradient-echo sequences typically have T2-weighting
C. The fat is bright in the spin-echo but not the gradient-echo sequences
D. The gradient-echo sequences deposit more energy onto the tissues
E. The spin-echo sequences require RF pulses to refocus magnetization, whereas, for the same purpose, gradient-echo sequences require refocusing gradients

Correct answer is E.

Spin-echo sequences typically include a 90° slice-selective pulse that puts the magnetization on the transverse plane, followed by (one or more) refocusing 180° pulses. Gradient-echo sequences typically use smaller flip angle pulses (<90°) and then use refocusing gradients to refocus magnetization on the transverse (*x*–*y*) plane. Gradient-echo sequences are typically much faster than spin-echo sequences and are used for cine images with high temporal resolution (multiple phases per cardiac cycle). The gradient-echo sequences can have more T1- or T2 (T2*)-weighting based on the flip angle used (smaller flip angles provide more T1-weighting) [2, 5]. Fat gives high signal (appears bright) in both spin-echo and gradient-echo sequences. Lastly, the energy deposited onto the tissues depends on the number of the RF pulses, which, in general, is greater in spin-echo sequences.

20. Which of the following may *not* be a gradient-echo sequence?

A. Steady-state free precession (SSFP)
B. Fast field-echo (FFE)
C. Echoplanar (EPI)
D. Inversion recovery (IR)
E. Time-of-flight (TOF)

Correct answer is D.

IR sequences provide heavy T1-weighting by first inverting the magnetization (with a 180° RF pulse) followed by a 90° RF pulse that brings the residual longitudinal magnetization into the transverse (*x*–*y*) plane, where it can be detected by the receiver RF coil. The time between the initial 180° pulse and the 90° pulse is the inversion time (TI). In CMR, the signal is usually refocused with a 180° pulse, as in a spin-echo sequence, although IR can also be combined with gradient-echo sequences [11].

21. Which of the following sequences can measure blood flow?

A. T1-weighted fast spin-echo sequences
B. T2-weighted fast spin-echo sequences
C. Phase-encoded sequences
D. IR sequences
E. Gadolinium-enhanced fast spin-echo sequences

Correct answer is C.

Phase-encoded sequences (also called phase-contrast [PC] or velocity-encoded [VENC] sequences) are gradient-echo sequences that can quantify the phase shift of the precession of protons that move inside a gradient magnetic field. This phase shift is proportional to the velocity of the protons. Thus, a velocity map can be obtained and superimposed on a magnitude image that can be spatially localized. Phase-encoded sequences are routinely used to quantify blood flow in the great vessels [11]. T1- and T2-weighted spin-echo and IR sequences (with or without contrast enhancement) are typically used to assess myocardial anatomy and for tissue characterization. T1- and T2-weighted sequences can also be used to distinguish between stationary and rapid blood flow, but are not quantitative.

22. Which of the following statements is correct regarding spin-echo sequences?

A. Selection of short repetition time (TR) and short echo time (TE) gives T1-weighting
B. Selection of short TR and short TE gives T2-weighting
C. Selection of long TR and long TE gives T1-weighting
D. Selection of long TR and long TE gives proton-density (PD)-weighting
E. Selection of long TR and short TE gives T2-weighting

Correct answer is A.

One of the advantages of spin-echo sequences is that they provide a clear contrast mechanism and can be modified to preferentially provide T1-, T2-, or PD-weighting [2, 11]. The following scheme describes how weighting depends on the technical parameters selected:

Short TR (450–850 ms) + short TE (10–30 ms) = T1-weighted
Long TR (2,000+ ms) + long TE (>60 ms) = T2-weighted
Long TR + short TE = PD-weighted

23. Which of the following statements regarding the RF energy used in CMR systems is correct?

A. The RF energy used for clinical CMR is too low to cause any harm
B. Examinations longer than 1 hour in duration pose significant risk because of tissue energy deposition, but shorter examinations are safe
C. The upper acceptable levels of RF energy tissue deposition depend on the tissue/organ imaged
D. The basic gradient-echo sequence deposits more RF energy to the tissues than the basic spin-echo approach
E. The interaction of the static magnetic field with the RF energy is more harmful than the RF energy would be alone

Correct answer is C.

The biologic effects of the RF energy inside a static magnetic field are the same as outside. The US Food and Drug Administration (FDA), Center for Devices and Radiological Health (CDRH) has set limits on the specific absorption rate (SAR) of RF energy in the body. The acceptable limits for energy deposition are different for the various organs and range from 3 W/kg averaged over the head for 10 min to 12 W/kg in any 1 g of tissue in the extremities for 15 min. CDRH guidance levels for patient SARs during CMR scans [12] are comparable to the maximum permissible exposure levels for controlled areas recommended by the American National Standards Institute/Institute of Electrical and Electronics Engineers (ANSI/IEEE) C95.1 (1992) [13], which are 0.4 W/kg averaged over the whole body, 8 W/kg for any 1 g of tissue, and 20 W/kg averaged over any 10 g of tissue in the extremities. The basic spin-echo sequence uses refocusing RF pulses, whereas the gradient-echo sequences uses refocusing gradients. Therefore, the deposited RF energy is greater for the basic spin-echo sequence than for the gradient-echo approach.

24. Which of the following parameters is responsible for nerve stimulation during a CMR examination?

A. The magnetic field (B_0)
B. The rate of change of the magnetic field (dB/dt)
C. The RF pulse amplitude
D. The RF pulse phase
E. None of the above

Correct answer is B.

Time-varying magnetic fields (dB/dt) induce electrical currents within the body, which, in turn, can cause nerve or muscle stimulation [14]. Peripheral neuromuscular stimulation can result in twitching, pain, and a startle reaction, all of which can cause discomfort and restlessness. The FDA/CDRH level of concern for dB/dt is 20 T/s [12, 15]. The routinely used static magnetic field (0.5–3 T) has no known biologic effects [16]. The CDRH has established a guidance level for static B_0 fields of 4 T, above which, MRI studies could present risk to patients [12, 15]. Excessive RF energy deposition may cause tissue injury and skin burns.

25. What is the effect of current gadolinium-based contrast agents on the T1-relaxation time of biologic tissues?

A. T1 increases after contrast administration
B. T1 decreases after contrast administration
C. T1 is not significantly affected
D. T1 increases in some sequences and decreases in others
E. The T1 changes proportionally to the field strength

Correct answer is B.

Gadolinium decreases the T1 of the tissues in which it is distributed [17–19]. Gadolinium is used as a positive contrast agent, to increase the signal of tissues that take up gadolinium (i.e., highly vascular or inflamed structures) and differentiate these tissues from those that do not take up gadolinium (i.e., avascular structures, clots, cysts, etc.). T1 is also dependent on the field strength and it decreases in higher field strengths.

26. Current gadolinium chelates (e.g., Gd-DTPA) that are commonly used as CMR contrast agents are:

A. Intracellular agents
B. Extracellular agents
C. 60% extracellular and 40% intracellular
D. 40 % intracellular and 60% extracellular
E. Extracellular for the first 5 minutes after administration and then intracellular

Correct answer is B.

Gadolinium chelates are relatively large molecules (molecular weight, 0.5–1 kDa), that do not cross the cell membranes of intact cells. After intravascular administration, these contrast agents rapidly diffuse from the intravascular to the extracellular (interstitial) space [18, 19].

27. Gadolinium-based contrast agents are typically used for tissue characterization in CMR. Which of the following is correct regarding these agents?

A. The likelihood for an allergic reaction is significantly higher compared with the iodinated contrast media typically used in CT scanning
B. The likelihood for an allergic reaction is similar to that reported for the iodinated contrast media typically used in CT scanning
C. The likelihood for an allergic reaction is significantly lower compared with the iodinated contrast media typically used in CT scanning
D. These agents have a similar nephrotoxic profile to the iodinated contrast agents
E. A central line is required for contrast administration

Correct answer is C.

Gadolinium-based contrast agents have a very low incidence of allergic reactions (~$1/10^4$) [20, 21]. This is significantly lower (at least one order of magnitude) than that reported for iodinated contrast agents (~1.6/1,000) [22]. Gadolinium contrast agents are not considered to be nephrotoxic, and can be safely administered even in patients with moderately impaired renal function without need for dose adjustment. Recently, a potentially lethal systemic disorder, called nephrogenic systemic sclerosis/nephrogenic fibrosing dermopathy, was described in patients with preexisting moderate to severe renal failure who received gadolinium-based agents, raising some concern regarding the use of these contrast media in this patient population [23–26]. Gadolinium contrast media are typically administered via a peripheral vein by hand or with a power injector.

28. Which of the following is a contraindication to CMR?

A. An aortic stent placed for coarctation
B. An implantable cardiac defibrillator (ICD)
C. An intrauterine device
D. An inferior vena cava filter placed for recurrent pulmonary embolisms
E. A coronary stent

Correct answer is B.

The presence of an ICD or a permanent pacemaker is considered a contraindication for any MRI scan, although, for CMR, several recent studies have demonstrated a good safety profile [27–29]. Issues with erroneous sensing or therapy delivery may be overcome by switching off the defibrillator, but problems may occur from the induction of currents (Eddie currents) or local heating at the tip of the ICD wire. There are also issues with the device's "memory" and other advanced software functions after the MRI scan is completed. Stents and filters are not contraindications for CMR, because these devices are made from stainless steel or non-ferromagnetic alloy. Intrauterine devices are usually made of copper and are also not contraindications for CMR.

29. A 70-year-old patient is referred for a CMR study. During the safety screening, the patient reports placement of a brain clip for an intracranial aneurysm 7 years ago. Three years ago, the patient had a shoulder MRI at another facility. Which of the following statements is correct?

A. It is not safe to perform the CMR study. Brain clip displacement will occur
B. It is definitely safe to perform the study. The patient had already an MRI that documented the safety of the examination
C. More information regarding the type of the clip should be obtained before proceeding with the CMR study
D. The patient can undergo the study so long as no EPI sequences are used
E. Performing the study in a 3-T system would be safer than in a 1.5-T system

Correct answer is C.

Intracranial aneurysm clips of various manufacturers have been shown to have small amounts of admixtures from metals that may be subject to attractive forces inside a strong magnetic field. Only titanium and titanium-alloy brain clips have been documented to be safe for MRI [30]. Intracranial aneurysm clips should be considered as a possible contraindication for CMR, and an apparently uneventful MRI study does not guarantee the safety of a subsequent study. The higher field systems are less safe, because the possible attractive forces would be even greater.

30. A patient with an artificial prosthetic valve is referred for CMR. What would you advise the referring physician regarding the safety of the examination at 1.5 T?

A. It is not safe to perform the examination because of the prosthetic valve
B. Most of the older valves (manufactured up to 2005) are not safe for CMR. However valves inserted after 2005 are CMR safe
C. Biologic valves are CMR safe but not mechanical valves
D. A chest X-ray should be performed first; if there is metal present, the CMR examination should not be performed
E. Both biologic and metallic cardiac valve prostheses are safe for CMR

Correct answer is E.

Cardiac prosthetic valves are generally safe for CMR for low (up to 1.5 T) magnetic fields [31]. There have been some theoretical concerns regarding very early Starr–Edwards valves (ball–cage) before series 6000. In higher field strengths (4.7 T), the CE Physio Ring (made from Elgiloy) seemed to develop an increasing magnetism on reentry into the MRI system, raising concerns regarding safety [32].

31. Why is it risky to perform a CMR examination in a non pacemaker-dependent patient with a permanent transvenous pacemaker?

A. Dislodging of the pacemaker generator may occur
B. Dislodging of the pacemaker lead(s) may occur
C. Permanent magnetization of the generator may cause malfunction after the CMR is performed
D. Inhibition of the generator may be inappropriate
E. Rapid stimulation may occur at the pacing lead tip

Correct answer is E.

The attractive force on the generator and the leads is not sufficiently strong to cause dislodging of either one. Malfunction of an implanted device after the MRI scan has been completed is a consideration for ICDs, but has not been an issue for pacemakers and particularly in non pacemaker-dependent patients. Similarly, although inappropriate inhibition of the pacemaker may occur during a CMR examination, this is usually not of concern in non pacemaker-dependent patients. Eddie currents and local heating in the pacemaker leads from the rapid gradient switching may cause rapid ventricular stimulation and possibly fatal arrhythmias [33].

32. A 60-year-old man is referred for a CMR study for evaluation of dyspnea. During his younger years, the patient had worked as a mechanic and metal welder. He has never had an MRI scan before. What is the most appropriate action?

A. Request orbit X-rays before proceeding with the CMR. Proceed only if there is no ocular shrapnel
B. Refer the patient for ophthalmology evaluation to exclude the presence of an intraocular foreign body
C. If the patient has no recollection of eye injury, proceed with the CMR examination
D. Start the CMR examination with a low-resolution image of the eyes and brain. Stop further imaging if there is any metal-related artifact
E. No reason to take any action based on the information provided. Proceed with the MRI examination as usual

Correct answer is A.

The patient's previous occupation makes it highly likely that shrapnel may have caused eye injury. Small metal pieces may remain for several years inside the eye with minimal symptomatology. Therefore, exclusion of intraocular metal objects is important and this is best performed with orbital X-rays or CT scanning [34]. Placing a patient with intraocular metal inside a strong magnetic field may cause dislodging of this metal and irreversible eye injury.

References

1. National Geophysical Data Center (NGDC). Earth's magnetic field calculators. http://www.ngdc.noaa.gov/seg/geomag/magfield.shtml.
2. van Geuns RJ, Wielopolski PA, de Bruin HG, et al. Basic principles of magnetic resonance imaging. *Prog Cardiovasc Dis*, 1999;42(2):149–156.
3. National Institute of Standards and Technology (NIST) NIfSaT. http://physics.nist.gov/.
4. Edelman RR and Warach S. Magnetic resonance imaging (1). *N Engl J Med*, 1993;328(10):708–716.
5. Longmore DB. The principles of magnetic resonance. *Br Med Bull*, 1989;45(4):848–880.
6. Schenck JF. Physical interactions of static magnetic fields with living tissues. *Prog Biophys Mol Biol*, 2005;87(2-3):185–204.
7. Bottomley PA, Foster TH, Argersinger RE, and Pfeifer LM. A review of normal tissue hydrogen NMR relaxation times and relaxation mechanisms from 1–100 MHz: dependence on tissue type, NMR frequency, temperature, species, excision, and age. *Med Phys*, 1984;11(4):425–448.
8. Gold GE, Han E, Stainsby J, Wright G, Brittain J, and Beaulieu C. Musculoskeletal MRI at 3.0 T: relaxation times and image contrast. AJR Am J Roentgenol, 2004;183(2):343–351.
9. Roussakis A, Baras P, Seimenis I, Andreou J, and Danias PG. Relationship of number of phases per cardiac cycle and accuracy of measurement of left ventricular volumes, ejection fraction, and mass. *J Cardiovasc Magn Reson*, 2004;6(4):837–844.
10. Fischer SE, Wickline SA, and Lorenz CH. Novel real-time R-wave detection algorithm based on the vectorcardiogram for accurate gated magnetic resonance acquisitions. *Magn Reson Med*, 1999;42(2):361–370.
11. Haacke EM, Li D, and Kaushikkar S. Cardiac MR imaging: principles and techniques. *Top Magn Reson Imaging*, 1995;7(4):200–217.
12. U.S. Department Of Health and Human Services FDA, Center for Devices and Radiological Health (CDRH). Guidance for the submission of premarket notifications for magnetic resonance diagnostic devices. http://www.fda.gov/cdrh/ode/mri340.pdf. 1998.
13. C95.1 ANSI/IEEE. IEEE Standard for Safety Levels with Respect to Human Exposure to Radio Frequency Electromagnetic Fields, 3 kHz to 300 GHz," ANSI/IEEE C95.1-1992 (Revision of ANSI C95.1-1982), Institute of Electrical and Electronics Engineers, Inc., Piscataway, NJ. 1992.
14. Schaefer DJ, Bourland JD, and Nyenhuis JA. Review of patient safety in time-varying gradient fields. *J Magn Reson Imaging*, 2000;12(1):20–29.
15. U.S. Department Of Health and Human Services FDA, Center for Devices and Radiological Health (CDRH). Guidance for industry and FDA staff. Criteria for significant risk investigations of magnetic resonance diagnostic devices. http://www.fda.gov/cdrh/ode/guidance/793.pdf. 2003.
16. Schenck JF. Safety of strong, static magnetic fields. *J Magn Reson Imaging*, 2000;12(1): 2–19.
17. Barnhart JL and Berk RN. Influence of paramagnetic ions and pH on proton NMR relaxation of biologic fluids. *Invest Radiol*, 1986;21(2):132–136.
18. Strich G, Hagan PL, Gerber KH, and Slutsky RA. Tissue distribution and magnetic resonance spin lattice relaxation effects of gadolinium-DTPA. *Radiology*, 1985;154(3):723–726.
19. Strijkers GJ, Mulder WJ, van Tilborg GA, and Nicolay K. MRI contrast agents: current status and future perspectives. *Anticancer Agents Med Chem*, 2007;7(3):291–305.
20. Kirchin MA and Runge VM. Contrast agents for magnetic resonance imaging: safety update. *Top Magn Reson Imaging*, 2003;14(5):426–435.
21. Li A, Wong CS, Wong MK, Lee CM, and Au Yeung MC. Acute adverse reactions to magnetic resonance contrast media—gadolinium chelates. *Br J Radiol*, 2006;79(941):368–371.
22. Caro JJ, Trindade E, and McGregor M. The risks of death and of severe nonfatal reactions with high- vs low-osmolality contrast media: a meta-analysis. *AJR Am J Roentgenol*, 1991;156(4):825–832.

23. Grobner T and Prischl FC. Gadolinium and nephrogenic systemic fibrosis. *Kidney Int*, 2007;72(3):260–264.
24. Broome DR, Girguis MS, Baron PW, Cottrell AC, Kjellin I, and Kirk GA. Gadodiamide-associated nephrogenic systemic fibrosis: why radiologists should be concerned. *AJR Am J Roentgenol*, 2007;188(2):586–592.
25. Karlik SJ. Gadodiamide-associated nephrogenic systemic fibrosis. *AJR Am J Roentgenol*, 2007;188(6):W584; author reply W585.
26. Sadowski EA, Bennett LK, Chan MR, et al. Nephrogenic systemic fibrosis: risk factors and incidence estimation. *Radiology*, 2007;243(1):148–157.
27. Roguin A, Zviman MM, Meininger GR, et al. Modern pacemaker and implantable cardioverter/defibrillator systems can be magnetic resonance imaging safe: in vitro and in vivo assessment of safety and function at 1.5 T. *Circulation*, 2004;110(5):475–482.
28. Shellock FG, Fischer L, and Fieno DS. Cardiac pacemakers and implantable cardioverter defibrillators: in vitro magnetic resonance imaging evaluation at 1.5-tesla. *J Cardiovasc Magn Reson*, 2007;9(1):21–31.
29. Martin ET, Coman JA, Shellock FG, Pulling CC, Fair R, and Jenkins K. Magnetic resonance imaging and cardiac pacemaker safety at 1.5-Tesla. *J Am Coll Cardiol*, 2004;43(7): 1315–1324.
30. Shellock FG, Tkach JA, Ruggieri PM, Masaryk TJ, and Rasmussen PA. Aneurysm clips: evaluation of magnetic field interactions and translational attraction by use of "long-bore" and "short-bore" 3.0-T MR imaging systems. *AJNR Am J Neuroradiol*, 2003;24(3):463–471.
31. Shellock FG. Magnetic resonance safety update 2002: implants and devices. *J Magn Reson Imaging*, 2002;16(5):485–496.
32. Edwards MB, Ordidge RJ, Hand JW, Taylor KM, and Young IR. Assessment of magnetic field (4.7 T) induced forces on prosthetic heart valves and annuloplasty rings. *J Magn Reson Imaging*, 2005;22(2):311–317.
33. Shinbane JS, Colletti PM, and Shellock FG. MR in patients with pacemakers and ICDs: Defining the issues. *J Cardiovasc Magn Reson*, 2007;9(1):5–13.
34. Boutin RD, Briggs JE, and Williamson MR. Injuries associated with MR imaging: survey of safety records and methods used to screen patients for metallic foreign bodies before imaging. *AJR Am J Roentgenol*, 1994;162(1):189–194.

2

General Cardiovascular Magnetic Resonance Imaging

Peter G. Danias, *Cardiovascular MRI: 150 Multiple-Choice Questions and Answers*

1. Anatomic and functional cardiovascular magnetic resonance imaging (CMR) requires:

A. Ability to perform long breath-holds (>15 s)
B. Weight <100 kg (220 lbs)
C. Sinus rhythm
D. Absence of coronary stents
E. Claustrophobia management

Correct answer is E.

CMR imaging no longer requires prolonged breath holding [1]. Patients of up to 230 kg (400 lb) may be imaged, although image quality may be suboptimal in the morbidly obese [2]. The presence of regular sinus rhythm is desirable for cardiac imaging but not mandatory. Stents cause local image artifacts but are not contraindication for CMR [3–5]. Claustrophobia management is essential before CMR is attempted.

2. In comparing CMR with other noninvasive imaging modalities, which of the following statements is correct?

A. The exposure to ionizing radiation with CMR is more than with a single chest X-ray, but considerably less than that of a chest computed tomography (CT) scan
B. The exposure to ionizing radiation with CMR is more than with a Tc-99 m myocardial perfusion single-photon emission computed tomography (SPECT) study, but considerably less than that of a TL-201 planar study
C. Because of high spatial and temporal resolution, CMR is better than echocardiography for evaluation of small and highly mobile structures
D. Because of the ability to perform volumetric imaging with high spatial and temporal resolution, CMR is the "gold standard" for measurement of ventricular volumes, mass, and ejection fraction
E. Coronary calcium detection is much better with CMR than with a multidetector CT (MDCT) scan

Correct answer is D.

CMR has no associated ionizing radiation exposure at all. CMR allows for volumetric imaging in any orientation and offers high spatial and temporal resolution. Measurements of right and left ventricular volumes, mass, and ejection fraction are highly accurate and reproducible, establishing CMR as the reference standard for these quantities [6–9]. CMR is not particularly good for evaluation of small and highly mobile structures (e.g., valve leaflets, vegetations, etc.), because the high resolution CMR requires ECG gating for acquisition of the entire image data set over several cardiac cycles. Highly mobile structures may not be at exactly the same position in several cardiac cycles and, thus, misregistration may occur, with subsequent image blurring. X-ray imaging (fluoroscopy and CT) are much better than CMR in visualizing coronary calcifications [10].

3. Which of the following statements comparing CMR with other noninvasive imaging technologies is correct?

A. Clinical CMR can image the coronary arteries with superior spatial resolution compared with 64-detector MDCT
B. Clinical CMR cine functional imaging has higher temporal resolution than M-mode echocardiography
C. CMR is better than transthoracic echocardiography in assessing valvular structure
D. Flow measurements by CMR are more reliable than those from transthoracic echocardiography in assessing calcific aortic valvular stenosis
E. Flow measurements by CMR are more reliable than those from transthoracic echocardiography in assessing aortic valvular insufficiency

Correct answer is E.

The in-plane spatial resolution of clinical CMR for coronary artery imaging is typically $1 \times 1\,mm^2$, with a slice thickness of 1.5 to 2.0mm [11]. Current 64-row MDCT technology can achieve imaging with isotropic voxels of $0.4 \times 0.4 \times 0.4\,mm^3$ [12]. However, CMR temporal resolution still remains better than that of MDCT. On the other hand, the temporal resolution of echocardiography (and particularly M-mode) is even higher (typically 1–5ms) [13]. CMR is unproven for assessing small structures that are rapidly moving (such as the cardiac valves or vegetations). CMR flow measurements are not always accurate for assessing the severity of valvular stenosis, because there are limitations on the phase encoding of high flow velocities [14]. CMR flow measurements are very accurate for quantitative measurement of valvular regurgitant lesions and compare favorably to semiquantitative echocardiographic data [15–17].

4. For which of the following applications CMR is *not* the gold standard?

A. Evaluation of anomalous coronary arteries
B. Assessment of infarcted myocardium
C. Measurement of left ventricular ejection fraction
D. Measurement of right ventricular end-diastolic volume
E. Assessment of coronary atherosclerosis

Correct answer is E.

CMR has been validated in phantom, experimental animal, and human studies as the most accurate technique to measure left and right ventricular volumes and ejection fraction [6, 7, 9, 18]. CMR can also visualize the origin and proximal course of the coronary arteries and is better than (or at least equivalent to) conventional contrast X-ray angiography for assessment of coronary anomalies [19, 20]. Cardiac CT with contrast enhancement can also accurately visualize the coronary anomalies, but the associated contrast load and X-ray radiation exposure may not be appropriate for younger patients. Delayed contrast-enhanced CMR can accurately assess the infarcted myocardium, with excellent correlation with pathology data [21–23]. CMR is still not able to reliably visualize coronary atherosclerosis and, therefore, cannot be considered the gold standard for this indication.

5. In a patient with atrial fibrillation and wide variability of the RR interval, who is undergoing CMR, which of the following statements is correct?

A. The left ventricular ejection fraction cannot be measured
B. The measured left ventricular ejection fraction grossly overestimates the systolic performance
C. The measured left ventricular ejection fraction correlates well with invasively measured values
D. The left ventricular mass cannot be measured
E. The myocardial viability cannot be assessed

Correct answer is C.

With significant RR variability, the diastolic period varies among different cardiac cycles. Systole, on the other hand, occurs usually at approximately 250 to 300 ms from the QRS complex and is less dependent on the heart rate than is diastole [24]. In a cine CMR study, the first phase to be obtained (starting on the QRS complex) is the end diastole. Systole and early diastole can be imaged and, thus, the end-diastolic volume and mass can be accurately measured. The end-systolic volume may be expected to slightly underestimate the actual systolic ventricular performance, because it will be the average of cycles with low(er) systolic performance occurring at cycles after a short RR interval (decreased preload, Frank Starling's law) with cycles with high(er) systolic performance occurring at cycles after long RR cycles (increased preload). Accordingly, the measured left ventricular ejection fraction may slightly underestimate the actual systolic performance. Despite these theoretical considerations, one study that specifically investigated measurements of left ventricular volumes and ejection fraction with prospective ECG-gated CMR and invasive contrast ventriculography in 26 patients with atrial fibrillation did not find significant discrepancy between the two methods [25]. Myocardial viability can be assessed both with delayed enhanced images (timed at systole) or with low-dose dobutamine administration, which will demonstrate the anticipated augmentation of systolic function, if viability is present.

6. Which of the following patients should *not* be assessed with CMR?

A. A 46-year-old patient with severe congestive heart failure, orthopnea, tachycardia, and low oxygen saturation (89% on a 100% O_2 face mask)
B. A 70-year-old patient with moderately severe aortic regurgitation, considered for aortic valve surgery
C. A 10-year-old patient with coarctation managed with an aortic stent 2 years ago

D. A woman with exertional syncope
E. A patient with coronary artery disease and severe left ventricular systolic dysfunction (ejection fraction 20%) who is being considered for revascularization

Correct answer is A.

The patient described in option A is unstable and likely to not tolerate supine positioning required for CMR. CMR is an appropriate test to quantitatively assess aortic regurgitation and precisely quantify left ventricular volumes and aortic dimensions [15–17, 26]. CMR is also appropriate for assessment of patients with coarctation [27, 28]. In the woman with exertional syncope, CMR can exclude the presence of hypertrophic cardiomyopathy, assess for anomalous coronary arteries, and evaluate for arrhythmogenic right ventricular dysplasia or other myocarditises/cardiomyopathies. Finally, CMR is an appropriate test to assess for the presence of myocardial viability in patients with severe left ventricular dysfunction considered for revascularization [18, 21].

7. A 25-year-old patient is referred for CMR. As soon as he is placed in the scanner, he becomes diaphoretic, his pulse increases to 160 beats per minute, and he complains of nausea and lightheadedness. The most appropriate approach would be to:

A. First place a peripheral intravenous line and then proceed with the study as planned
B. Administer a mild sedative (e.g., a short acting benzodiazepine) orally, place nasal prongs for supplemental oxygen, and then proceed with the study
C. Stop the study. Administer oxygen via nasal cannula and immediately obtain a medical evaluation of the patient and, if needed, a 12-lead ECG
D. Stop the study. Discharge the patient to home with instructions to contact his physician
E. Ask the patient if he is willing to proceed with the study, and if the patient agrees, proceed as planned

Correct answer is C.

Hemodynamic instability is a contraindication for CMR imaging. This patient may have had a panic attack inside the CMR scanner, but medical causes of the tachycardia and possible hypotension (lightheadedness, diaphoresis, and nausea) have to be evaluated and addressed as needed. Presumptive treatment for anxiety would be inappropriate, as would be discharging the patient to home without appropriate medical evaluation and treatment.

8. Figure 2.1 shows a diastolic (left panel) and a systolic (right panel) image from a cine study at the 2-chamber (long axis) orientation. Identify the structures on the diastolic frame.

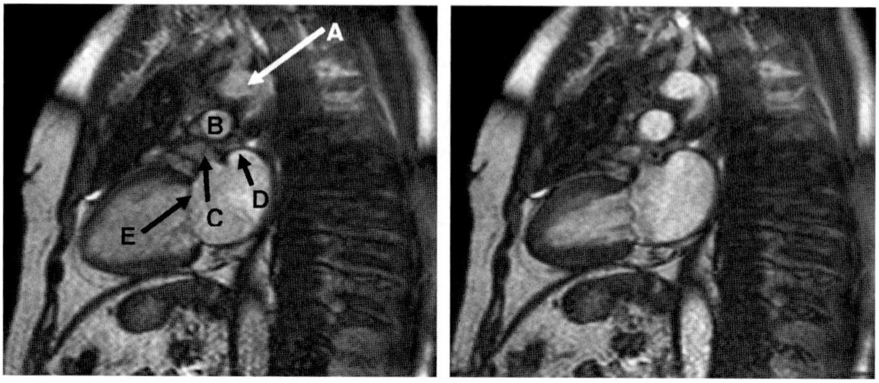

A. A = aortic arch; B = right pulmonary artery; C = left upper pulmonary vein; D = left atrial appendage; and E = anterior leaflet of the mitral valve
B. A = aortic arch; B = left pulmonary artery; C = left upper pulmonary vein; D = left atrial appendage; and E = anterior leaflet of the mitral valve
C. A = aortic arch; B = right pulmonary artery; C = left atrial appendage; D = left upper pulmonary vein; and E = anterior leaflet of the mitral valve
D. A = aortic arch; B = left pulmonary artery; C = left atrial appendage; D = left upper pulmonary vein; and E = anterior leaflet of the mitral valve
E. A = aortic arch; B = left pulmonary artery; C = left atrial appendage; D = left upper pulmonary vein; and E = posterior leaflet of the mitral valve

Correct answer is D.

The left atrial appendage is an anterior structure of the left atrium, whereas the pulmonary veins are posterior structures (Fig. 2.2). *Ao*, aorta; *LPA*, left pulmonary artery; *LAAp*, left atrial appendage; *LUPV*, left upper pulmonary vein; *AntMV*, anterior leaflet of the mitral valve.

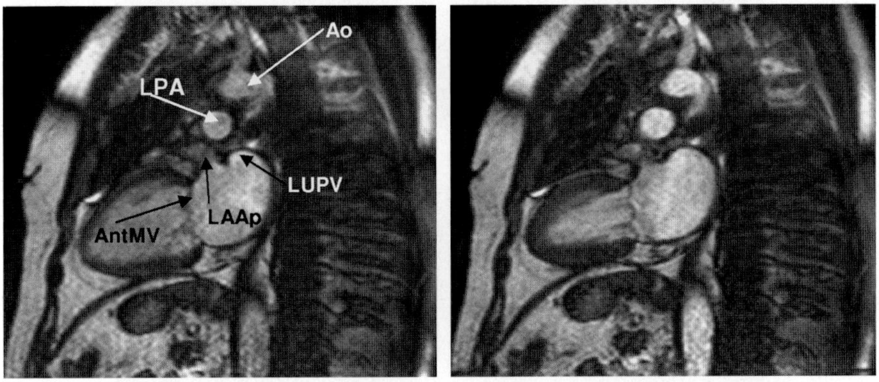

9. Figure 2.3 is a single frame from a gadolinium-enhanced CMR angiogram, obtained in the coronal orientation. What is the likely diagnosis?

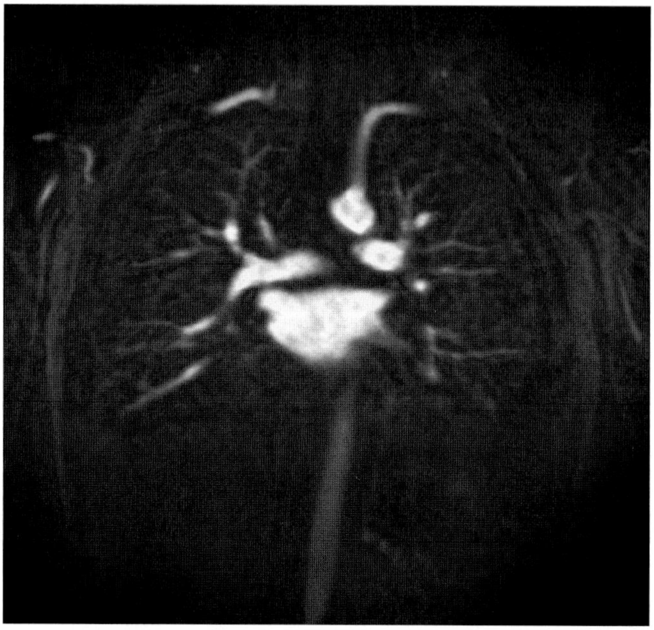

A. Anomalous pulmonary venous return
B. Transposition of the great arteries status post (s/p) Mustard correction
C. Hypoplasia of the left pulmonary artery
D. Patent ductus arteriosus
E. Normal anatomy

Correct answer is E.

Figure 2.4 has all structures labeled appropriately and represents normal anatomy. The slice is posteriorly located in the thoracic cavity, as is evident by the visualization of the four pulmonary veins entering into the left atrium (which typically involves the posterior left atrial wall) and the descending thoracic aorta, a structure of the posterior mediastinum. *AA*, aortic arch; *DAo*, descending thoracic aorta; *LLPV*, left lower pulmonary vein; *LPA*, left pulmonary artery; *LSbclvA*, left subclavian artery; *LUPV*, left upper pulmonary vein; *RLPV*, right lower pulmonary vein; *RPA*, right pulmonary artery; *RUPV*, right upper pulmonary vein.

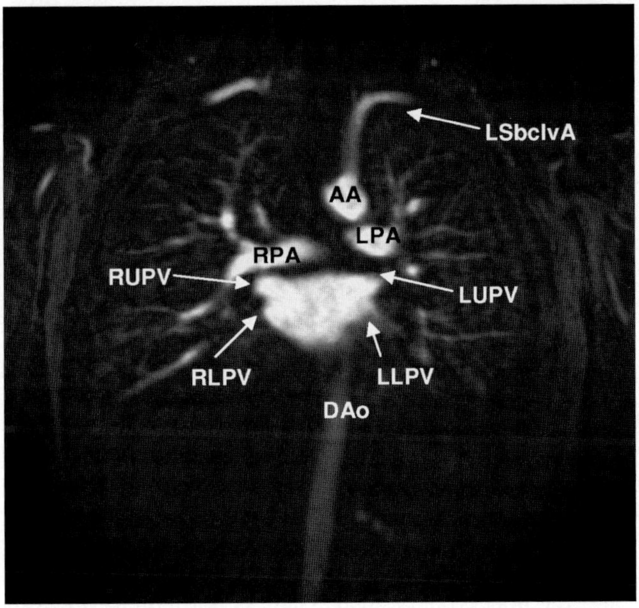

10. Figure 2.5 was obtained during a coronary MR angiogram in a patient evaluated for possible anomalous takeoff of the right coronary artery. The orientation of the image plane is parallel to the atrioventricular groove.

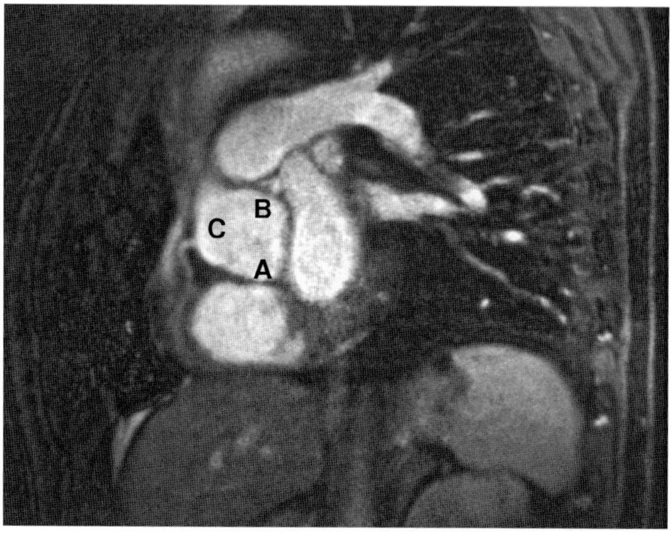

Which of the following statements is correct regarding this study?

A. C indicates the right coronary cusp. There is anomalous takeoff of the right coronary artery from the left coronary cusp
B. C indicates the left coronary cusp. There is normal takeoff of the right coronary artery from the right coronary cusp
C. B indicates the noncoronary cusp. There is normal takeoff of the right coronary artery from the right coronary cusp
D. B indicates the left coronary cusp. There is normal takeoff of the right coronary artery from the right coronary cusp
E. It is not possible from this image to identify the coronary cusps and to ascertain whether the right coronary artery has a normal origin or not

Correct answer is D.

Figure 2.6 has all cardiac structures labeled. *LA*, left atrium; *PA*, pulmonary artery; *RA*, right atrium. The angulated arrow shows the intraatrial septum. The noncoronary cusp is the one located against the intra-atrial septum and, thus, cusp *A* is the noncoronary one. The right coronary cusp is located anteriorly (*C*), and, thus, *B* is the left cusp. The coronary artery shown (*white arrow*) originates at the right coronary cusp and courses in the right atrioventricular groove. This is the normal takeoff and proximal course of the right coronary artery. The left coronary artery originates from the left cusp (*B*) and its proximal segment (in cross section) is indicated with the *black arrow*.

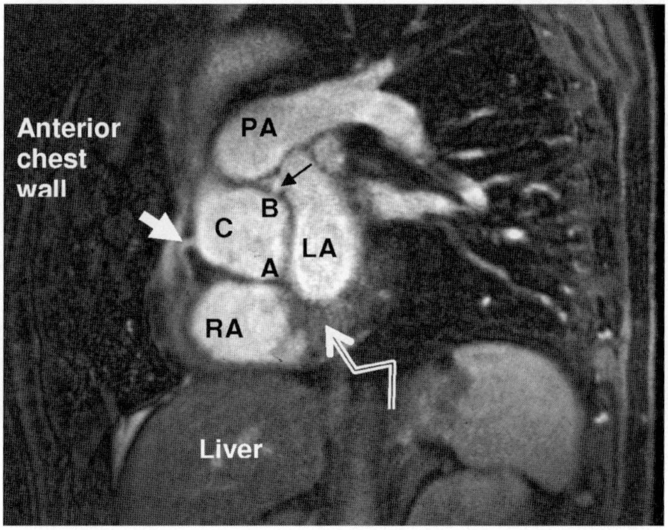

11. Figure 2.7 is a single frame from a functional CMR study obtained at the short axis orientation. What structure is indicated by the arrows?

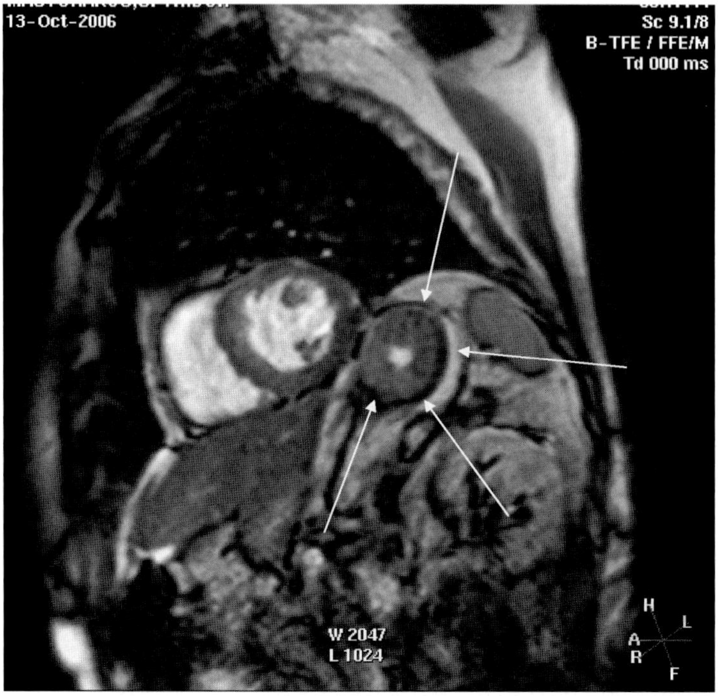

A. Stomach
B. Left ventricular aneurysm
C. Transplanted heart
D. Artifact
E. Aortic aneurysm

Correct answer is A.

In this short-axis image (Fig. 2.8) the left and right ventricles (*LV* and *RV*, respectively) are easily identified. The *white arrowheads* indicate the left hemidiaphragm. The liver and stomach (*S*) are identified as subdiaphragmatic structures. No artifact would present like this. The aorta is usually not inside the field-of-view in the short-axis orientation.

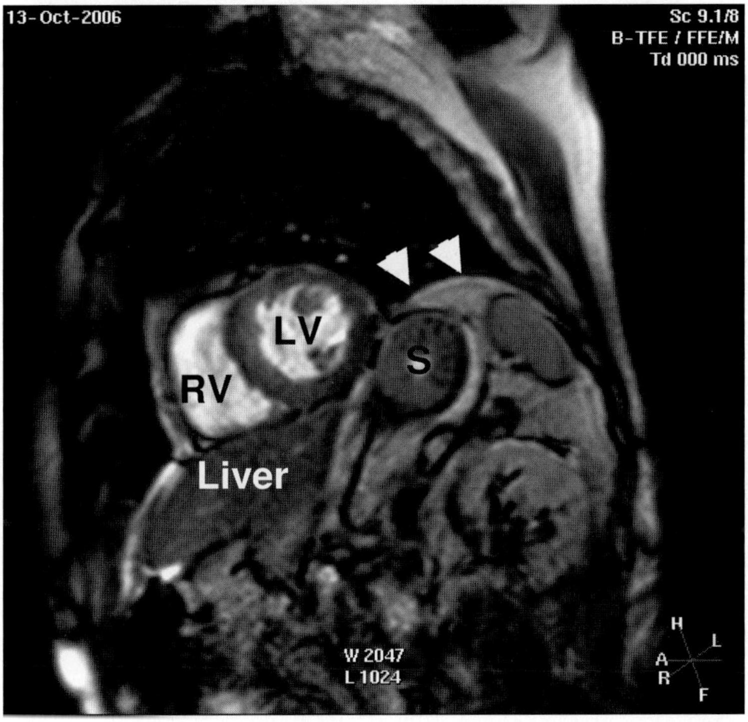

12. Figure 2.9 is a transverse slice obtained with a black blood sequence at the base of the heart. Which of the following options best identifies the structures that are numbered on the image?

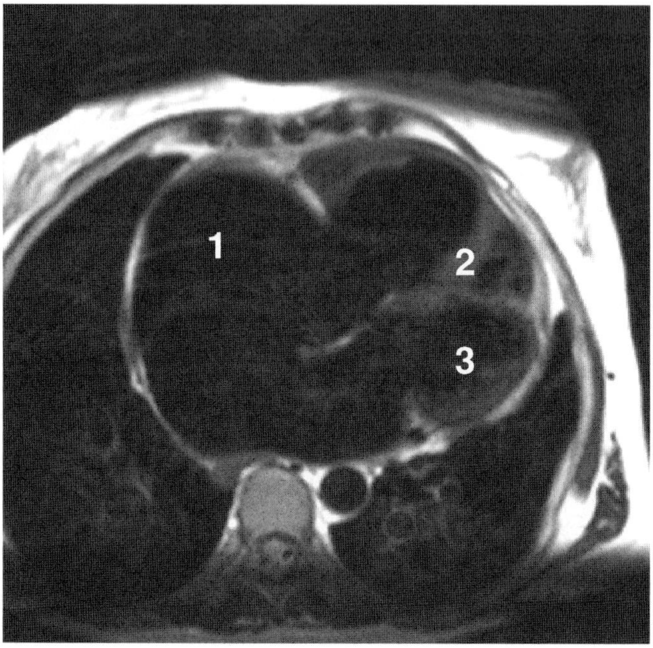

A. 1 = right atrium; 2 = intraventricular septum; 3 = left ventricle
B. 1 = left atrium; 2 = left ventricle; 3 = right ventricle
C. 1 = right atrium; 2 = moderator band; 3 = left ventricle
D. 1 = coronary sinus; 2 = intraventricular septum; 3 = left ventricle
E. 1 = common atrium; 2 = intraventricular septum; 3 = left ventricle

Correct answer is C.

Figure 2.10 is obtained from a patient with a large secundum atrial septal defect (*arrows*). The right and left atria (*ra* and *la*, respectively) are significantly dilated. The right ventricle (*RV*) is dilated and the moderator band (*mb*) is prominent. The left ventricle (*LV*) is small compared with the other cardiac chambers. The intraventricular septum (*ivs*) is also indicated.

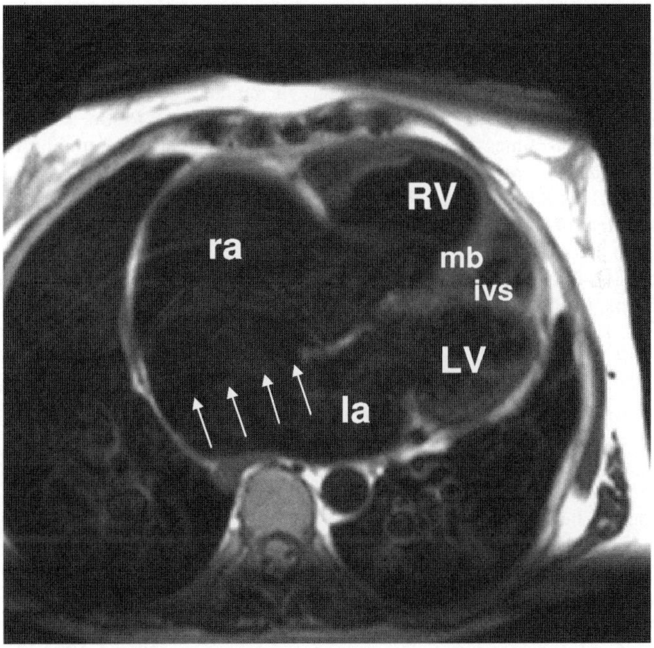

References

1. Danilouchkine MG, Westenberg JJ, Lelieveldt BP, and Reiber JH. Accuracy of short-axis cardiac MRI automatically derived from scout acquisitions in free-breathing and breath-holding modes. *Magma*, 2005;18(1):7–18.
2. Danias PG, Tritos NA, Stuber M, Kissinger KV, Salton CJ, and Manning WJ. Cardiac structure and function in the obese: a cardiovascular magnetic resonance imaging study. *J Cardiovasc Magn Reson*, 2003;5(3):431–438.
3. Gerber TC, Fasseas P, Lennon RJ, et al. Clinical safety of magnetic resonance imaging early after coronary artery stent placement. J Am Coll Cardiol, 2003;42(7):1295–1298.
4. Schroeder AP, Houlind K, Pedersen EM, Thuesen L, Nielsen TT, and Egeblad H. Magnetic resonance imaging seems safe in patients with intracoronary stents. *J Cardiovasc Magn Reson*, 2000;2(1):43–49.
5. Strohm O, Kivelitz D, Gross W, et al. Safety of implantable coronary stents during 1H-magnetic resonance imaging at 1.0 and 1.5 T. *J Cardiovasc Magn Reson*, 1999;1(3):239–245.
6. Alfakih K, Reid S, Jones T, and Sivananthan M. Assessment of ventricular function and mass by cardiac magnetic resonance imaging. *Eur Radiol*, 2004;14(10):1813–1822.
7. Marcu CB, Beek AM, and Van Rossum AC. Cardiovascular magnetic resonance imaging for the assessment of right heart involvement in cardiac and pulmonary disease. Heart Lung Circ, 2006;15(6):362–370.
8. Myerson SG, Bellenger NG, and Pennell DJ. Assessment of left ventricular mass by cardiovascular magnetic resonance. *Hypertension*, 2002;39(3):750–755.
9. Pujadas S, Reddy GP, Weber O, Lee JJ, and Higgins CB. MR imaging assessment of cardiac function. *J Magn Reson Imaging*, 2004;19(6):789–799.
10. Berman DS, Hachamovitch R, Shaw LJ, et al. Roles of nuclear cardiology, cardiac computed tomography, and cardiac magnetic resonance: assessment of patients with suspected coronary artery disease. *J Nucl Med*, 2006;47(1):74–82.
11. Manning WJ, Nezafat R, Appelbaum E, Danias PG, Hauser TH, and Yeon SB. Coronary Magnetic Resonance Imaging. *Cardiol Clin*, 2007;25(1):141–170.
12. Hoffmann U, Ferencik M, Cury RC, and Pena AJ. Coronary CT angiography. *J Nucl Med*, 2006;47(5):797–806.
13. Carerj S, Micari A, Trono A, et al. Anatomical M-mode: an old-new technique. *Echocardiography*, 2003;20(4):357–361.
14. Sondergaard L, Hildebrandt P, Lindvig K, et al. Valve area and cardiac output in aortic stenosis: quantification by magnetic resonance velocity mapping. *Am Heart J*, 1993;126(5):1156–1164.
15. Chatzimavroudis GP, Oshinski JN, Franch RH, Walker PG, Yoganathan AP, and Pettigrew RI. Evaluation of the precision of magnetic resonance phase velocity mapping for blood flow measurements. *J Cardiovasc Magn Reson*, 2001;3(1):11–19.
16. Gelfand EV, Hughes S, Hauser TH, et al. Severity of mitral and aortic regurgitation as assessed by cardiovascular magnetic resonance: optimizing correlation with Doppler echocardiography. *J Cardiovasc Magn Reson*, 2006;8(3):503–507.
17. Ley S, Eichhorn J, Ley-Zaporozhan J, et al. Evaluation of aortic regurgitation in congenital heart disease: value of MR imaging in comparison to echocardiography. *Pediatr Radiol*, 2007;37(5):426–436.
18. Marcu CB, Beek AM, and van Rossum AC. Clinical applications of cardiovascular magnetic resonance imaging. *Cmaj*, 2006;175(8):911–917.
19. Danias PG, Stuber M, McConnell MV, and Manning WJ. The diagnosis of congenital coronary anomalies with magnetic resonance imaging. *Coron Artery Dis*, 2001;12(8):621–626.
20. Varghese A, Keegan J, and Pennell DJ. Cardiovascular magnetic resonance of anomalous coronary arteries. *Coron Artery Dis*, 2005;16(6):355–364.
21. Isbell DC and Kramer CM. Magnetic resonance for the assessment of myocardial viability. *Curr Opin Cardiol*, 2006;21(5):469–472.

22. Kim DH, Choi SI, Chang HJ, Choi DJ, Lim C, and Park JH. Delayed hyperenhancement by contrast-enhanced magnetic resonance imaging: Clinical application for various cardiac diseases. *J Comput Assist Tomogr*, 2006;30(2):226–232.
23. Vogel-Claussen J, Rochitte CE, Wu KC, et al. Delayed enhancement MR imaging: utility in myocardial assessment. *Radiographics*, 2006;26(3):795–810.
24. Greenfield JC, Jr., Harley A, Thompson HK, and Wallace AG. Pressure-flow studies in man during atrial fibrillation. *J Clin Invest*, 1968;47(10):2411–2421.
25. Hundley WG, Meshack BM, Willett DL, et al. Comparison of quantitation of left ventricular volume, ejection fraction, and cardiac output in patients with atrial fibrillation by cine magnetic resonance imaging versus invasive measurements. *Am J Cardiol*, 1996;78(10):1119–1123.
26. Wyttenbach R, Bremerich J, Saeed M, and Higgins CB. Integrated MR imaging approach to valvular heart disease. *Cardiol Clin*, 1998;16(2):277–294.
27. Didier D, Saint-Martin C, Lapierre C, et al. Coarctation of the aorta: pre and postoperative evaluation with MRI and MR angiography; correlation with echocardiography and surgery. *Int J Cardiovasc Imaging*, 2006;22(3-4):457–475.
28. Riehle TJ, Oshinski JN, Brummer ME, et al. Velocity-encoded magnetic resonance image assessment of regional aortic flow in coarctation patients. *Ann Thorac Surg*, 2006;81(3):1002–1007.

3

Valvular Heart Disease

Peter G. Danias, *Cardiovascular MRI: 150 Multiple-Choice Questions and Answers*

1. In Fig. 3.1, the steady-state free precession (SSFP) cine cardiovascular magnetic resonance imaging (CMR) scans are diastolic (*A*) and systolic (*B*) frames of a cine loop at the left ventricular outflow tract of a young patient with a murmur. What is the diagnosis?

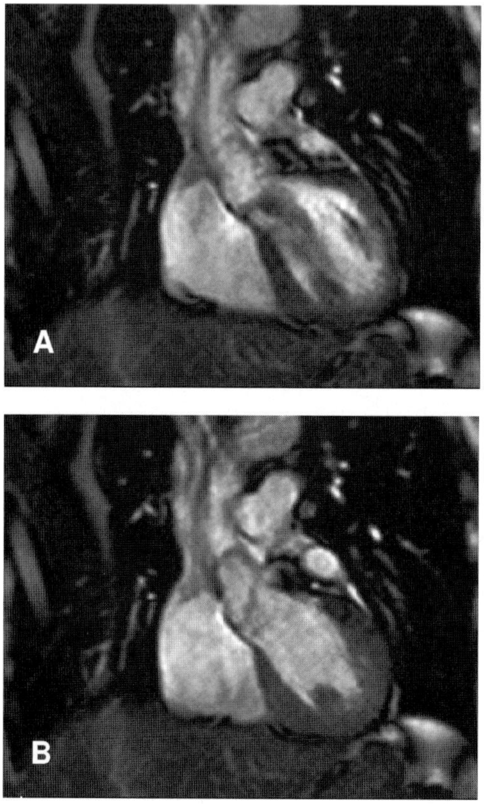

A. Severe aortic valve stenosis
B. Subvalvular aortic stenosis
C. Pulmonic valve stenosis
D. Aortic valve insufficiency
E. Pulmonary valve insufficiency

Correct answer is D.

In Fig. 3.2A (diastolic frame), there is a signal void in the left ventricular outflow tract (*arrows*). This is consistent with aortic regurgitation [1–5]. The size of the jet does not translate into severity of the valvular insufficiency, because it depends on many technical parameters and mainly on the echo time (TE) of the imaging sequence that was used [3]. There is no evidence of severe aortic stenosis (systolic signal void from high velocities in the aortic root), or subvalvular aortic stenosis (systolic signal void in the left ventricular outflow tract). The pulmonary valve is not visualized in these frames.

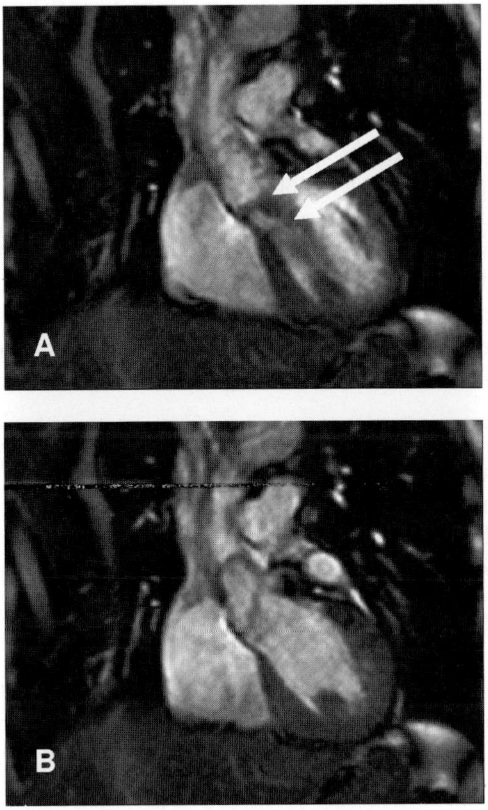

2. A patient with rheumatic heart disease undergoes CMR scanning. The following measurements are obtained:

Left ventricular end-diastolic volume: 160 mL
Left ventricular end-diastolic volume: 60 mL
Aortic root systolic forward flow: 80 mL
Aortic valve regurgitant fraction: 15%

What is the calculated mitral valve regurgitant fraction?

A. 5%
B. 10%
C. 20%
D. 30%
E. 40%

Correct answer is C.

During systole, the heart ejects blood forward in the aorta, and, if mitral valve regurgitation is present, backward into the left atrium. Therefore, left ventricular stroke volume equals aortic systolic forward flow plus mitral regurgitant flow. The left ventricular stroke volume is the end-diastolic minus the end-systolic volume.

Accordingly, in this case, the left ventricular stroke volume is $160 - 60 = 100$ mL, and the mitral regurgitant flow is $100 - 80 = 20$ mL. The mitral valve regurgitant fraction is the mitral regurgitant flow divided by the left ventricular stroke volume, which, in this case, is $20/100 \times 100\%$, i.e., 20%.

3. A 36-year-old man is noted to have a new murmur. Transthoracic echocardiography demonstrated a small highly mobile structure on the anterior mitral valve leaflet. The primary physician wants to refer this patient for a CMR scan. What would you advise the referring physician regarding the clinical usefulness of CMR for the suspected pathology?

A. CMR has definite advantages for diagnosis of endocarditis and is superior to transesophageal echocardiography for this purpose
B. CMR can usually identify small and highly mobile vegetations because it has high spatial and temporal resolution
C. CMR has little value in demonstrating vegetations that are highly mobile, but has potential value for evaluating complications of endocarditis
D. Contrast administration would be helpful to separate between vegetation and clot
E. CMR has greater sensitivity than blood cultures for detection of subacute bacterial endocarditis

Correct answer is C.

For ECG-gated sequences, small structures need to be in exactly the same position over time (over several cardiac cycles) to be visualized. This is why CMR is not particularly good for detecting pathology in small or thin and highly mobile structures (e.g., cardiac valves, vegetations, etc.). Real-time sequences allow for imaging of fast-moving structures without the need to return to the same position in consecutive cardiac cycles, but the current spatial resolution of real-time techniques is in the order of 3 to 4 mm, rather inadequate to image fine structures [6, 7]. CMR has been reported to be able to assess certain complications of endocarditis [8–11]. Valvular regurgitation can be quantified for all four cardiac valves with a fairly high degree of accuracy. Abscess formation may also be possible to visualize by CMR, although this does not constitute an established indication for CMR imaging. For the reasons described above, CMR has lower sensitivity for detection of bacterial endocarditis than either blood cultures or transesophageal echocardiography. Contrast administration would not be helpful to separate between vegetation and clot, because both structures are avascular and, thus, do not take up contrast.

4. In Fig. 3.3, *A* and *B* are systolic magnitude and phase images, respectively, from a phase-contrast study at the root of the pulmonary artery. The diagram in *C* represents the pulmonic flow data, derived from the automated analysis of the phase-contrast study. Which of the following statements is correct?

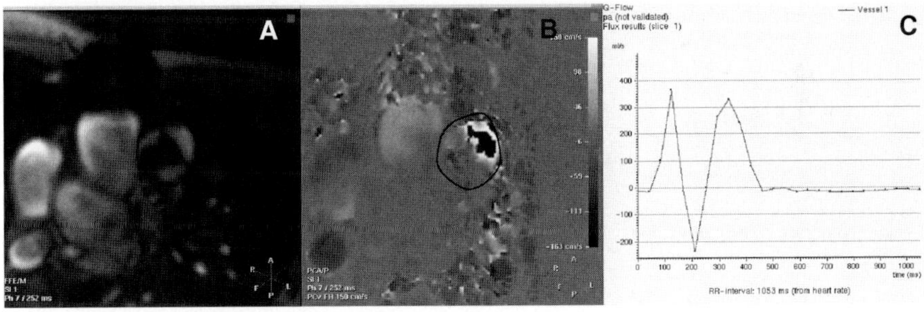

A. There is mid-systolic reversal of blood flow
B. There is significant flow deceleration during systole caused by subvalvular stenosis
C. There is pulmonic valve leaflet prolapse
D. There is no significant pulmonic insufficiency
E. There is artifact in the study that does not allow any conclusions to be drawn regarding the pulmonic valve function

Correct answer is D.

The flow analysis demonstrates an apparent flow reversal in the main pulmonary artery (Fig. 3.4C, *white curved arrow*), which is artifactual. The high velocities that occur during ejection in this patient are outside the range used for phase encoding in this scan [12], and a phenomenon similar to echocardiographic aliasing occurs (Fig. 3.4B, *black arrow*). It is, therefore, not possible from this image to measure the ejection velocities or to assess the presence of pulmonic valve stenosis. It is also not possible from this image to calculate accurately the forward blood flow. In diastole, however, the blood flow velocities are within the phase-encoding range, and, thus, an assessment regarding the presence of pulmonic valvular insufficiency can be made. In this case, there is no significant pulmonic insufficiency, demonstrated by the absence of negative flow values (under the zero line in the diagram) in diastole (Fig. 3.4C, *small black arrows*).

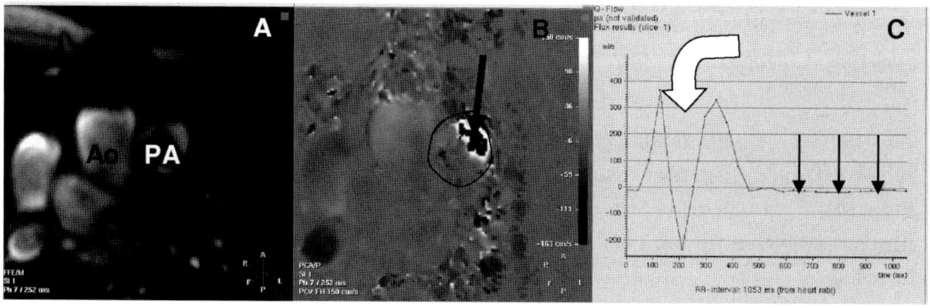

5. Figure 3.5 shows (*A*) diastolic and (*B*) systolic frames from a cine study obtained at the plane of the aortic valve in a patient with murmur.

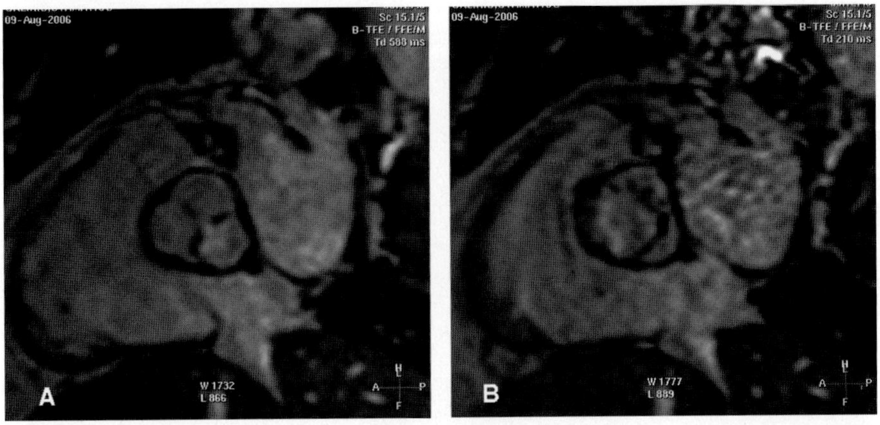

Which of the following statements is *not* correct?

A. The aortic valve is trileaflet
B. This image is obtained with a white blood sequence
C. It is unlikely that the patient has a significant intra-atrial septal defect
D. It is very likely that the patient has a significant ventricular septal defect
E. It is unlikely that the patient has severe aortic stenosis

Correct answer is D.

Figure 3.6A demonstrates a trileaflet aortic valve with good coaptation of the three cusps. The right (R), left (L) and noncoronary (NC) cusps are indicated. This white blood image also demonstrates normal diameter of the right ventricular outflow tract (RVOT), which is smaller than the aortic valve annulus, arguing against a hemodynamically significant intracardiac left-to-right shunt. Finally, it is unlikely that the patient has severe aortic stenosis, as demonstrated by the good opening of the valve in the systolic frame (white-out area, Fig. 3.6B).

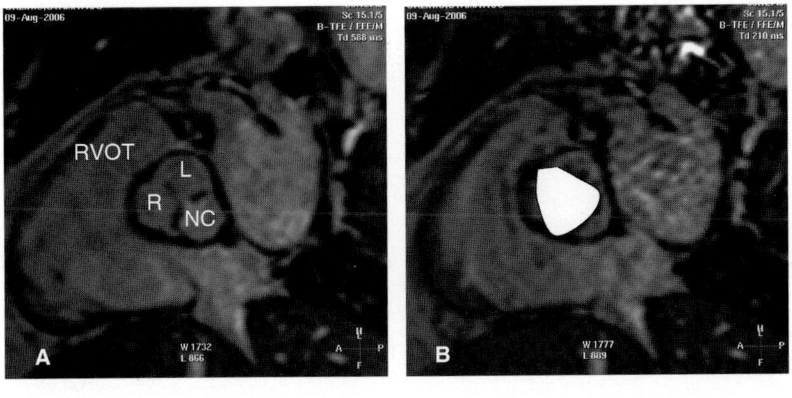

6. The data in Fig. 3.7 were obtained from analysis of a flow scan at a plane perpendicular to the aortic root in a patient with a murmur. What is the likely diagnosis?

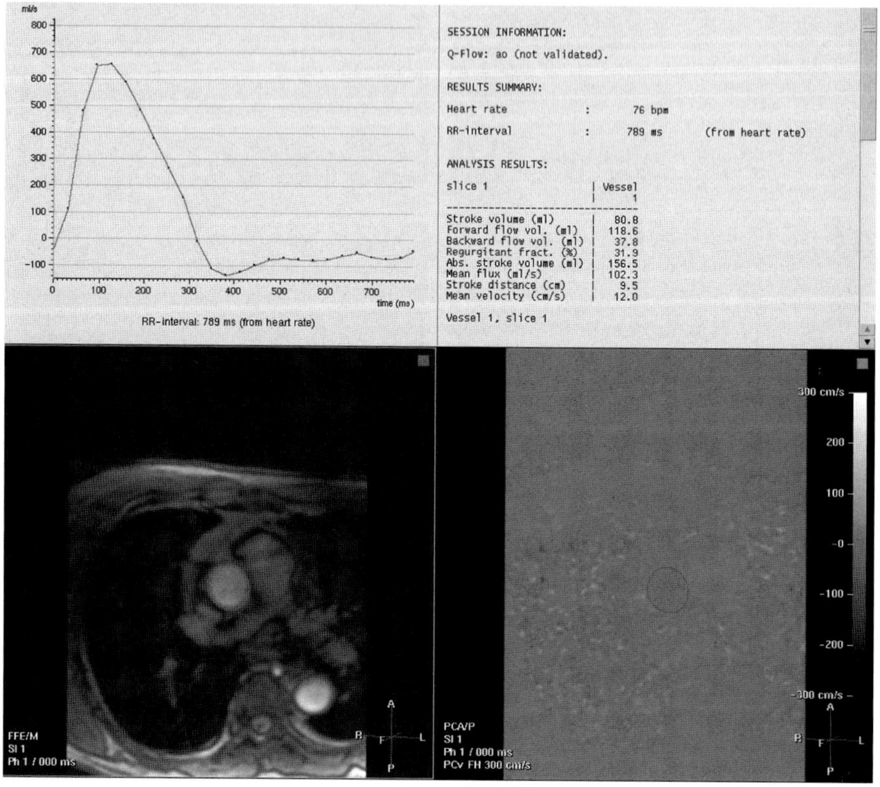

A. Aortic stenosis
B. Aortic regurgitation
C. Aortic root dissection
D. Severe mixed aortic disease (stenosis and regurgitation)
E. Coarctation

Correct answer is B.

The graph on the *upper left panel* in Fig 3.8 demonstrates negative flows during diastole (shaded area, curve under the zero line). This is suggestive of aortic regurgitation. In fact, the data analysis presented in the *right upper panel* in Fig 3.8, quantify this regurgitation as moderately severe (regurgitant fraction 32%). The pulmonary valve is not examined in this orientation, although the magnitude and phase scans (*lower left* and *right panels*, respectively) do not suggest significant pulmonary valve pathology. There is no evidence of increased velocities (absence of signal void in the magnitude image at the left lower panel in Fig. 3.8, or aliasing in the phase image at the right lower panel in Fig 3.8) at the aortic root or the descending thoracic aorta to suggest the diagnoses of aortic stenosis and coarctation, respectively.

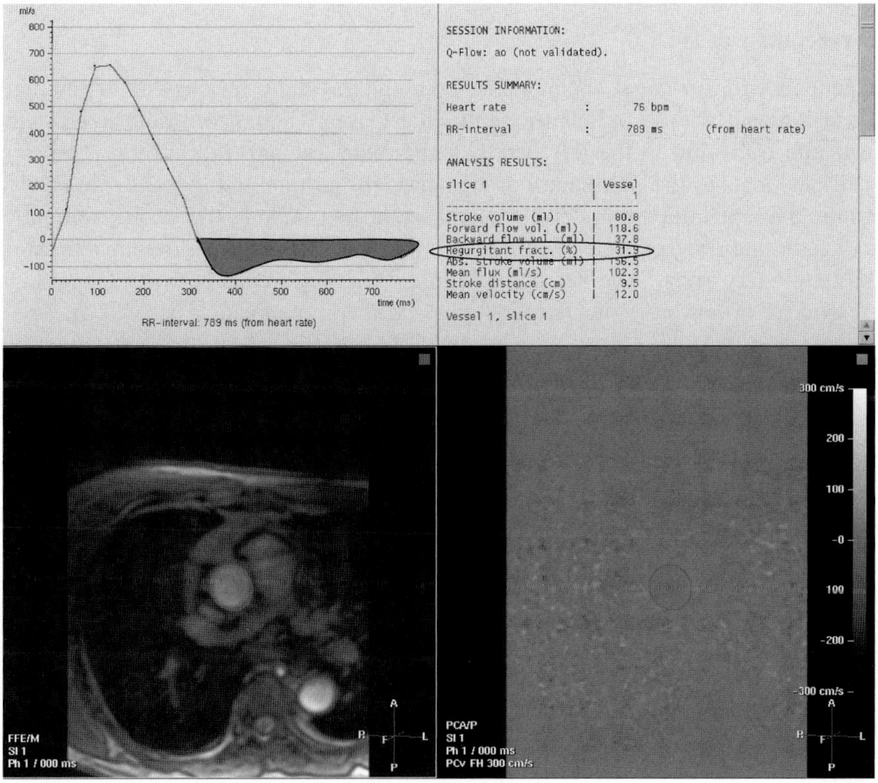

7. In a patient with atrioventricular septal defect (atrioventricular [AV] canal), which of the following statements is correct?

A. The left-to-right flow through the defect can be calculated by measuring the flow in the ascending aorta and the left ventricular stroke volume
B. The left-to-right flow through the defect can be calculated by measuring the flow in the pulmonary artery trunk and the right ventricular stroke volume
C. The left-to-right flow through the defect can be calculated by measuring the outflow in the pulmonary artery trunk and the inflow through the inferior and superior vena cava
D. The left-to-right flow through the defect can be calculated by measuring the flow in the ascending aorta and pulmonary artery trunk
E. The flow through the defect cannot be accurately measured

Correct answer is D.

In patients with AV canal, the blood of the both atria and ventricles mixes and there is usually insufficiency of the atrioventricular valves. The left ventricle ejects to the aorta and backward to the left atrium, right ventricle, and right atrium. The right ventricle ejects to the pulmonary artery, the right atrium, and, possibly, to the left atrium. The quantities that can be easily quantified include the stroke volume of both right and left ventricles and the ejection and net forward flow into the aorta and pulmonary artery. The net shunt volume is the difference between Qp and Qs, irrespective of how complicated the left-to-right communication is [13, 14].

8. The following measurements are obtained in a patient with tetralogy of Fallot who underwent a Blalock–Taussig shunt 2 years ago:

Left ventricular stroke volume: 58 ml
Aortic net forward flow: 50 ml
Right ventricular stroke volume: 40 ml
Pulmonary artery net forward flow: 35 ml

If we know that there are no aortopulmonary collateral vessels and no functioning patent ductus arteriosus, what is the flow through the Blalock–Taussig shunt?

A. 23 ml
B. 15 ml
C. 10 ml
D. 5 ml
E. There is no flow—the shunt is occluded

Correct answer is B.

The Blalock–Taussig shunt is a surgically created connection between the subclavian artery and pulmonary artery [15]. The net blood flow to the aortic root equals to the net pulmonic flow plus the shunt flow. Thus, the shunt flow is the difference between the aortic and pulmonic flow, i.e., 50 – 35 = 15 ml. In this patient, it is obvious that the shunt is not occluded, because the Qp/Qs = 35/50 = 0.7.

9. With phase encoding CMR, which of the following statements is *not* correct?

A. Aortic stenosis can be quantitatively assessed
B. The difference between systolic and diastolic coronary artery flow is a reliable measure of atherosclerosis
C. Mitral regurgitation can be measured both directly and indirectly
D. In patients with isolated mitral valve insufficiency and no other valvular abnormalities, mitral regurgitation can be calculated from the volumetric study of the left and right ventricles
E. Mitral regurgitation is best measured indirectly from the left heart volume and aortic flow data

Correct answer is B.

Phase contrast CMR is particularly good for measurement of relatively low blood flow velocities. With high velocities, phase wrapping (conceptually similar to echocardiographic aliasing) can occur and the flow measurements may become unreliable. Thus, special care must be made to set the appropriate velocity encoding range to directly measure the high flow velocities of mitral regurgitation and severe aortic stenosis [16–19]. Mitral regurgitation is best measured indirectly, by subtracting the forward systolic aortic flow (obtained from a phase-encoded study at the aortic root) from the left ventricular stroke volume (obtained from the volumetric cine study by applying Simpson's rule) [20, 21]. In patients with isolated mitral regurgitation, the difference between the left and right ventricular stroke volume is the mitral regurgitant volume [21]. Coronary sinus flow reserve has been assessed as a measure of coronary atherosclerosis.

10. What is the use of phase-contrast sequences for evaluation of the severity of coarctation?

A. To obtain a precise measurement of the aortic diameter at the site of stenosis
B. To provide an accurate measurement of the pressure gradient at the site of maximal stenosis
C. To assess the aortic valve insufficiency
D. To assess the left ventricular hypertrophy that is associated with the increased arterial blood pressure
E. To provide an indirect measure of collateral flow by quantifying the aortic blood flow proximal and distal to the site of maximal stenosis

Correct answer is E.

The dimensions of the aorta are best obtained with anatomic images (e.g., T1-weighted sequences) and not functional flow images. The pressure gradient at the site of stenosis may be measured by the phase-encoded sequences [22], but, commonly, there is flow turbulence, and the flow velocities may be too high for CMR to accurately measure [23]. Although aortic valve insufficiency in patients with coarctation may be accurately measured, this is not a measure of aortic stenosis at the site of coarctation. Left ventricular hypertrophy cannot be measured with flow studies (phase-encoded sequences). By measuring the flow proximal and distal to the site of stenosis, the collateral blood flow may be indirectly quantified as their numerical difference. The collateral flow is an indirect measure of the severity of aortic lumen stenosis [24, 25].

11. Figure 3.9 shows diastolic (*A*) and systolic (*B*) images from a cine CMR study in the 3-chamber orientation. Which of the following statements best describes the findings of this study?

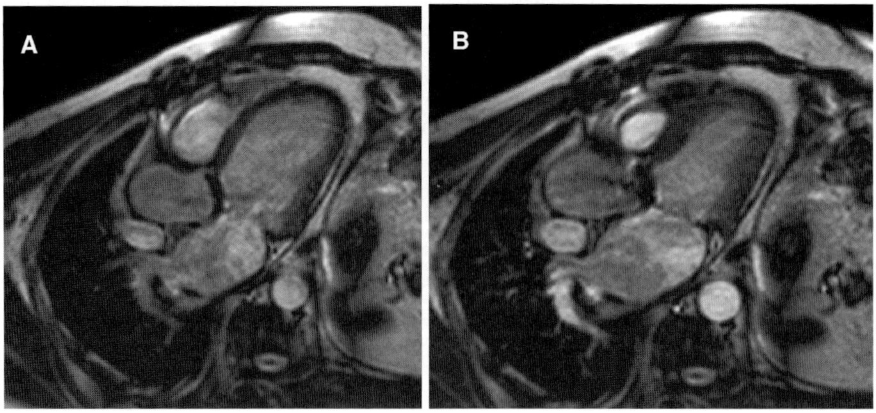

A. There is aortic valve calcification with significant regurgitation
B. There is aortic valve calcification with significant stenosis
C. There is aortic valve calcification with significant mixed disease
D. There is a metallic prosthetic valve with some aortic regurgitation
E. There is a metallic prosthetic valve with severe aortic stenosis

Correct answer is D.

The *white arrows* in Fig. 3.10A indicate the susceptibility artifact from the sternal wires, suggesting a previous cardiothoracic operation. The *black arrow* indicates the diastolic jet at the left ventricular outflow tract, suggesting some aortic regurgitation. The size of the jet does not imply the severity of the valvular insufficiency, because it largely depends on technical factors of the acquisition sequence (namely the echo time [TE]) [3]. The *open white arrows* (*B*) indicate the susceptibility artifact (complete signal loss) that the metallic aortic valve causes. The signal void at the aortic root (*white arrowhead*) is caused by turbulent flow during the ventricular ejection phase, which invariably occurs with prosthetic aortic valves.

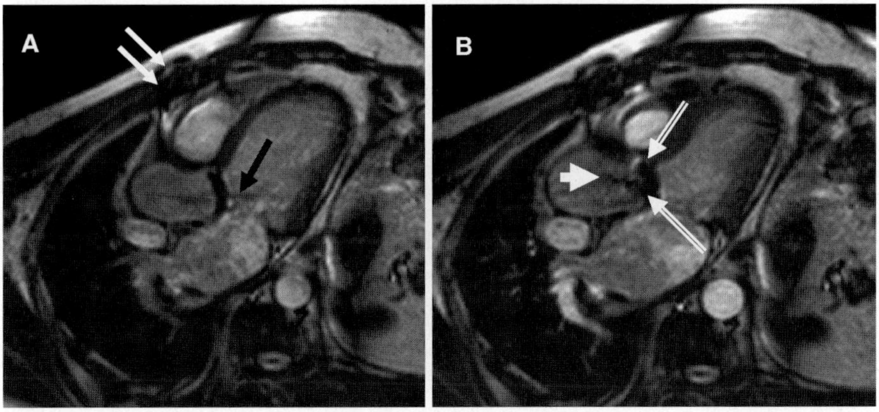

12. A 35-year-old patient with endocarditis develops severe dyspnea (Fig. 3.11). A CMR study demonstrates normal left ventricular systolic function. The calculated stroke volume of the left ventricle is 130 ml. A phase-contrast study is performed and blood flow is measured at the aortic root. The flow analysis is displayed in the graph in Fig. 3.11.

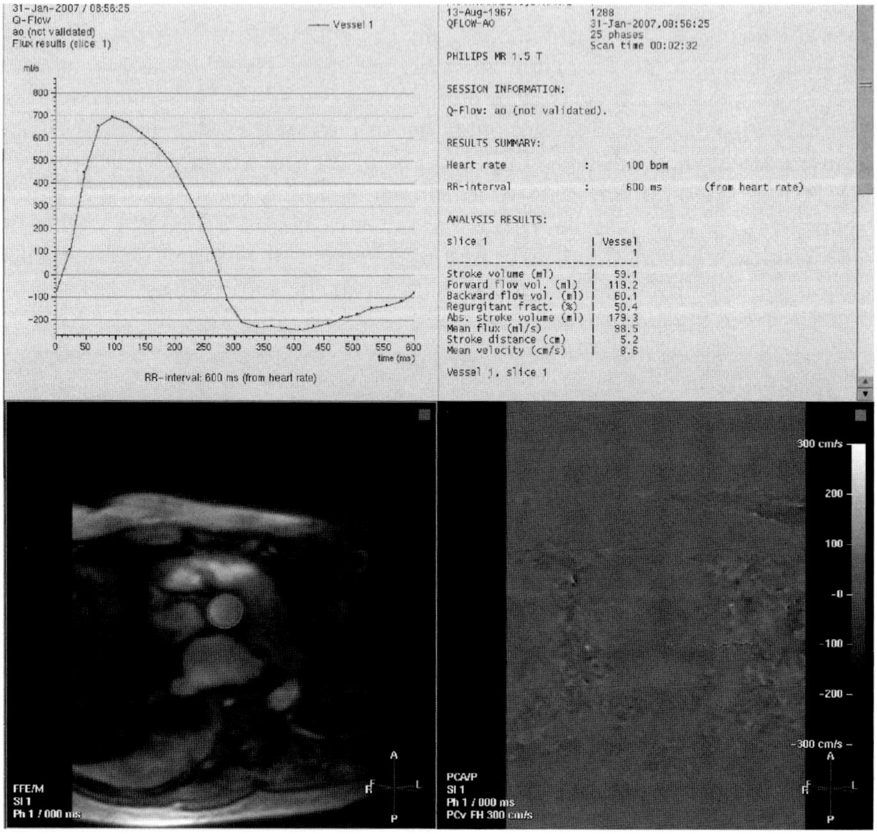

What is the most likely cause of the dyspnea?

A. Severe mitral regurgitation
B. Severe aortic regurgitation
C. Mild aortic regurgitation
D. Severe aortic and mitral valve regurgitation
E. Mild aortic and mitral regurgitation

Correct answer is B.

The flow analysis at the aortic root demonstrates severe aortic regurgitation (Fig. 3.12, *shaded grey area* under the zero line, indicating backward flow) and a regurgitant fraction of 50%. The mitral valve regurgitant volume in this case would be 130 ml (left ventricular stroke volume) minus 119 ml (aortic systolic flow), i.e., 11 ml, corresponding to a regurgitant fraction of approximately 8% (i.e., mild mitral regurgitation). The right pleural effusion noted on the magnitude image (Fig. 3.12, *white arrow*) is most likely caused by congestive left heart failure.

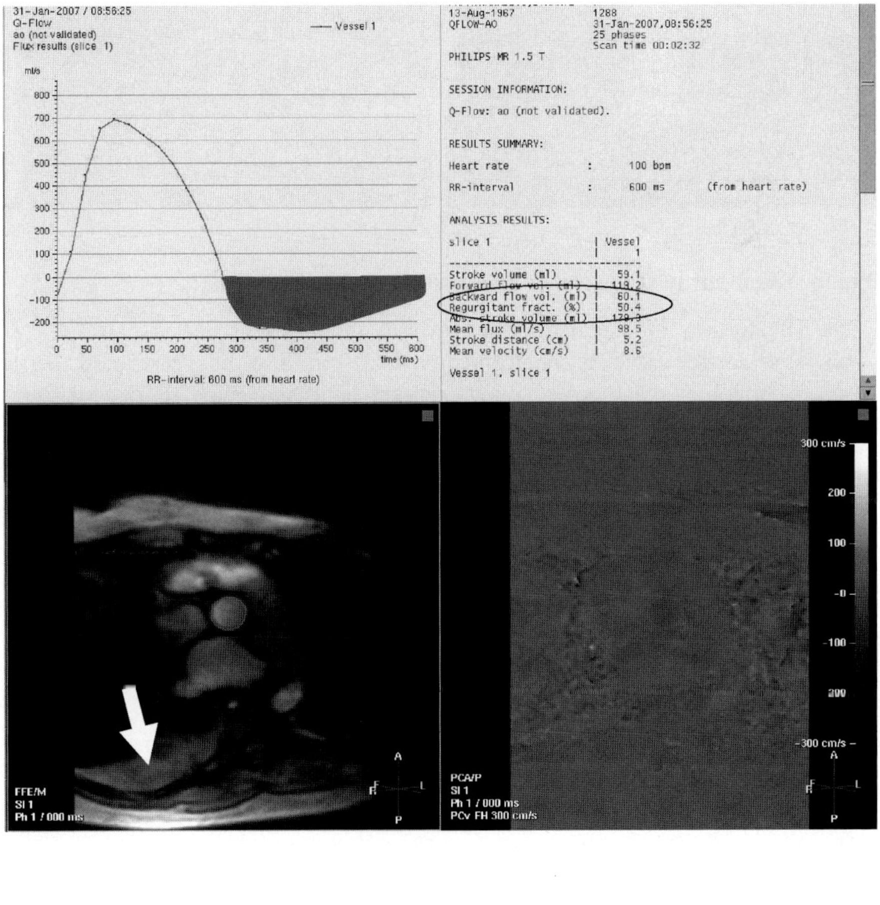

13. Figure 3.13 shows diastolic (*A*) and systolic (*B*) images from a cine study obtained at the root of the aorta.

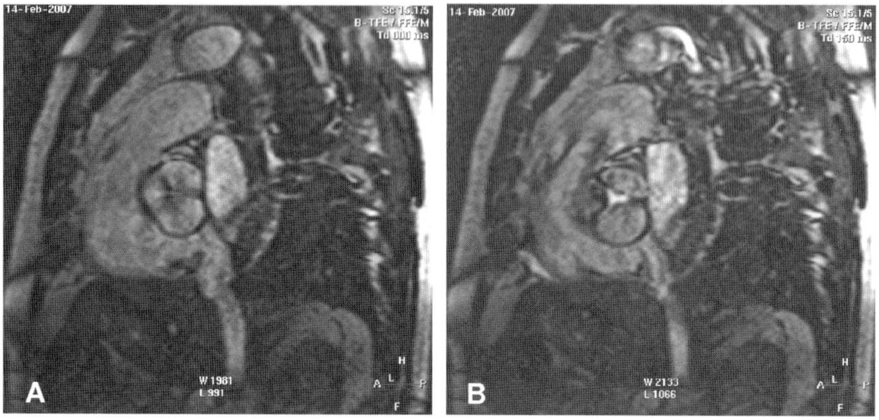

Which statement best describes the aortic valve in Fig. 3.13?

A. The aortic valve is trileaflet but severely incompetent
B. The aortic valve is anatomically bicuspid and has restricted leaflet excursion
C. The aortic valve is functionally bicuspid and has restricted leaflet excursion
D. The aortic valve is trileaflet and has restricted leaflet excursion
E. The aortic valve is anatomically and functionally normal

Correct answer is D.

The aortic valve is trileaflet and the three cusps are labeled in Fig. 3.14 (*L*, left; *R*, right; *NC*, noncoronary). There is restriction of the excursion of the leaflets, evident by the small area of the orifice (Fig. 3.14B, *whited out area* in the systolic frame). In both frames, there is signal loss at the site of coaptation of the three leaflets (Fig. 3.14A, *arrows*) suggesting degenerative changes and calcification of the commissures. CMR planimetry of the aortic valve orifice has been shown to provide an accurate estimation of the degree of aortic valve stenosis [26, 27], although some have reported overestimation of the valve area with CMR [28]. In Fig. 3.14A, coaptation at end diastole seems to be intact, arguing against severe aortic valve insufficiency.

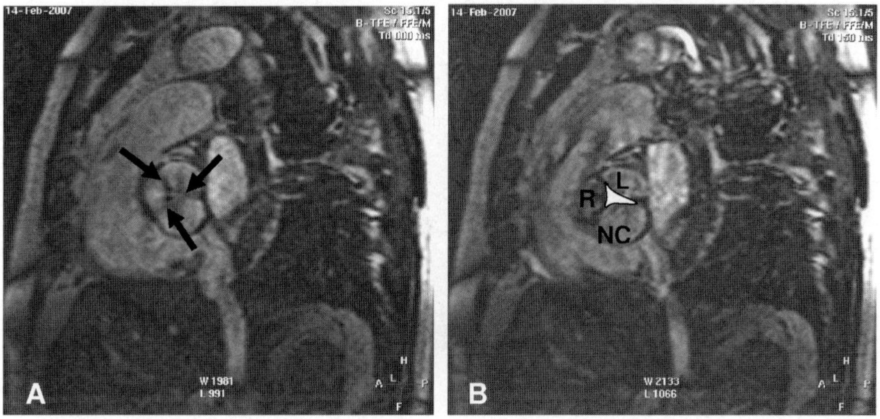

14. A young woman is referred for a CMR evaluation of acute severe aortic insufficiency. Figure 3.15 shows a transverse slice from a SSFP bright blood sequence (mixed weighting, more T2).

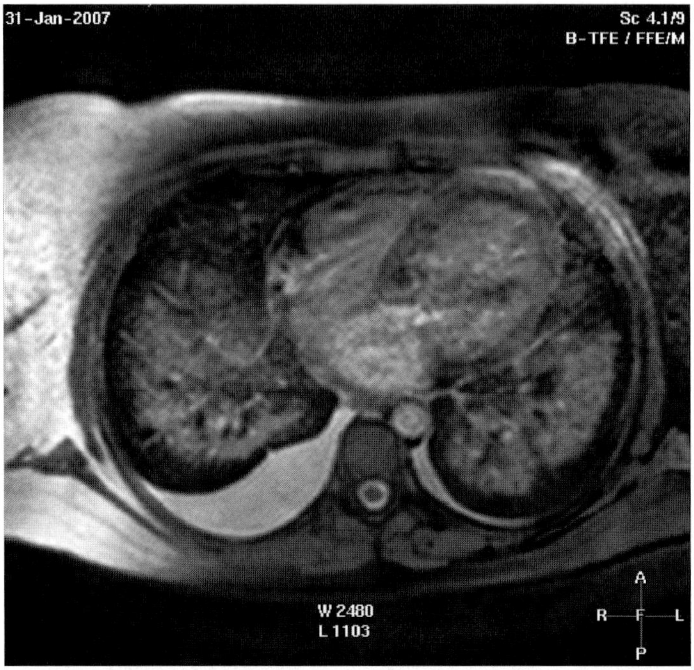

Which is an appropriate statement based on Fig. 3.15?

A. The patient has septic emboli to the right lung with associated right pleural effusion
B. The patient has a right sided pulmonary embolus with associated right pleural effusion
C. The patient has severe heart failure
D. The patient has severe right-sided lobar pneumonia
E. There is severe image artifact in the lung tissue

Correct answer is C.

The image demonstrates severe parenchymal pulmonary congestion and tissue edema with increased signal inside the lungs, and mostly at the (dependent) posterior lung fields. There are also bilateral pleural effusions, right more than left. Lastly, there is left ventricular dilation. These findings suggest the presence of severe congestive heart failure, also corroborated by the clinical information provided. Unilateral pathology would not explain the pathologic appearance of both lungs and the bilateral pleural effusions. No lung-related artifact is seen in this image.

References

1. Didier D. Assessment of valve disease: qualitative and quantitative. *Magn Reson Imaging Clin N Am*, 2003;11(1):115–134, vii.
2. Higgins CB, Wagner S, Kondo C, Suzuki J, and Caputo GR. Evaluation of valvular heart disease with cine gradient echo magnetic resonance imaging. *Circulation*, 1991;84(3 Suppl):I198–207.
3. Suzuki J, Caputo GR, Kondo C, and Higgins CB. Cine MR imaging of valvular heart disease: display and imaging parameters affect the size of the signal void caused by valvular regurgitation. *AJR Am J Roentgenol*, 1990;155(4):723–727.
4. Wagner S, Auffermann W, Buser P, et al. Diagnostic accuracy and estimation of the severity of valvular regurgitation from the signal void on cine magnetic resonance images. *Am Heart J*, 1989;118(4):760–767.
5. Krombach GA, Kuhl H, Bucker A, et al. Cine MR imaging of heart valve dysfunction with segmented true fast imaging with steady state free precession. *J Magn Reson Imaging*, 2004;19(1):59–67.
6. Guttman MA, Kellman P, Dick AJ, Lederman RJ, and McVeigh ER. Real-time accelerated interactive MRI with adaptive TSENSE and UNFOLD. *Magn Reson Med*, 2003;50(2):315–321.
7. Weiger M, Pruessmann KP, and Boesiger P. Cardiac real-time imaging using SENSE. SENSitivity Encoding scheme. *Magn Reson Med*, 2000;43(2):177–184.
8. Carpenter JL. Perivalvular extension of infection in patients with infectious endocarditis. *Rev Infect Dis*, 1991;13(1):127–138.
9. Hwang SW, Yucel EK, and Bernard S. Aortic root abscess with fistula formation. *Chest*, 1997;111(5):1436–1438.
10. Miller SW, Palmer EL, Dinsmore RE, and Brady TJ. Gallium-67 and magnetic resonance imaging in aortic root abscess. *J Nucl Med*, 1987;28(10):1616–1619.
11. Saghir S, Ivey TD, Kereiakes DJ, and Mazur W. Anterior mitral valve leaflet aneurysm due to infective endocarditis detected by cardiac magnetic resonance imaging. *Rev Cardiovasc Med*, 2006;7(3):157–159.
12. Underwood SR, Firmin DN, Rees RS, and Longmore DB. Magnetic resonance velocity mapping. *Clin Phys Physiol Meas*, 1990;11 Suppl A:37–43.
13. Gutierrez FR, Siegel MJ, Fallah JH, and Poustchi-Amin M. Magnetic resonance imaging of cyanotic and noncyanotic congenital heart disease. *Magn Reson Imaging Clin N Am*, 2002;10(2):209–235.
14. Wang ZJ, Reddy GP, Gotway MB, Yeh BM, and Higgins CB. Cardiovascular shunts: MR imaging evaluation. *Radiographics*, 2003;23 Spec No:S181–194.
15. Ullom RL, Sade RM, Crawford FA, Jr., Ross BA, and Spinale F. The Blalock-Taussig shunt in infants: standard versus modified. *Ann Thorac Surg*, 1987;44(5):539–543.
16. Friedrich MG, Schulz-Menger J, Poetsch T, Pilz B, Uhlich F, and Dietz R. Quantification of valvular aortic stenosis by magnetic resonance imaging. *Am Heart J*, 2002;144(2):329–334.
17. Westenberg JJ, Doornbos J, Versteegh MI, et al. Accurate quantitation of regurgitant volume with MRI in patients selected for mitral valve repair. *Eur J Cardiothorac Surg*, 2005;27(3):462–466; discussion 467.
18. Nayak KS, Hu BS, and Nishimura DG. Rapid quantitation of high-speed flow jets. *Magn Reson Med*, 2003;50(2):366–372.
19. Waters EA, Caruthers SD, and Wickline SA. Correlation analysis of stenotic aortic valve flow patterns using phase contrast MRI. *Ann Biomed Eng*, 2005;33(7):878–887.
20. Hundley WG, Li HF, Willard JE, et al. Magnetic resonance imaging assessment of the severity of mitral regurgitation. Comparison with invasive techniques. *Circulation*, 1995;92(5):1151–1158.
21. Kon MW, Myerson SG, Moat NE, and Pennell DJ. Quantification of regurgitant fraction in mitral regurgitation by cardiovascular magnetic resonance: comparison of techniques. *J Heart Valve Dis*, 2004;13(4):600–607.

22. Mohiaddin RH, Kilner PJ, Rees S, and Longmore DB. Magnetic resonance volume flow and jet velocity mapping in aortic coarctation. *J Am Coll Cardiol*, 1993;22(5):1515–1521.
23. Eichhorn JG, Fink C, Delorme S, Hagl S, Kauczor HU, and Ulmer HE. Magnetic resonance blood flow measurements in the follow-up of pediatric patients with aortic coarctation—a re-evaluation. *Int J Cardiol*, 2006;113(3):291–298.
24. Julsrud PR, Breen JF, Felmlee JP, Warnes CA, Connolly HM, and Schaff HV. Coarctation of the aorta: collateral flow assessment with phase-contrast MR angiography. *AJR Am J Roentgenol*, 1997;169(6):1735–1742.
25. Pujadas S, Reddy GP, Weber O, Tan C, Moore P, and Higgins CB. Phase contrast MR imaging to measure changes in collateral blood flow after stenting of recurrent aortic coarctation: initial experience. *J Magn Reson Imaging*, 2006;24(1):72–76.
26. Reant P, Lederlin M, Lafitte S, et al. Absolute assessment of aortic valve stenosis by planimetry using cardiovascular magnetic resonance imaging: comparison with transesophageal echocardiography, transthoracic echocardiography, and cardiac catheterisation. *Eur J Radiol*, 2006;59(2):276–283.
27. Schlosser T, Malyar N, Jochims M, et al. Quantific of aortic valve stenosis in MRI-comparison of steady-state free precession and fast low-angle shot sequences. *Eur Radiol*, 2007;17(5): 1284–1290.
28. Debl K, Djavidani B, Seitz J, et al. Planimetry of aortic valve area in aortic stenosis by magnetic resonance imaging. *Invest Radiol*, 2005;40(10):631–636.

4

Diseases of the Myocardium and Pericardium

Peter G. Danias, *Cardiovascular MRI: 150 Multiple-Choice Questions and Answers*

1. Fig. 4.1 is a short-axis midventricular T1-weighted black blood image.

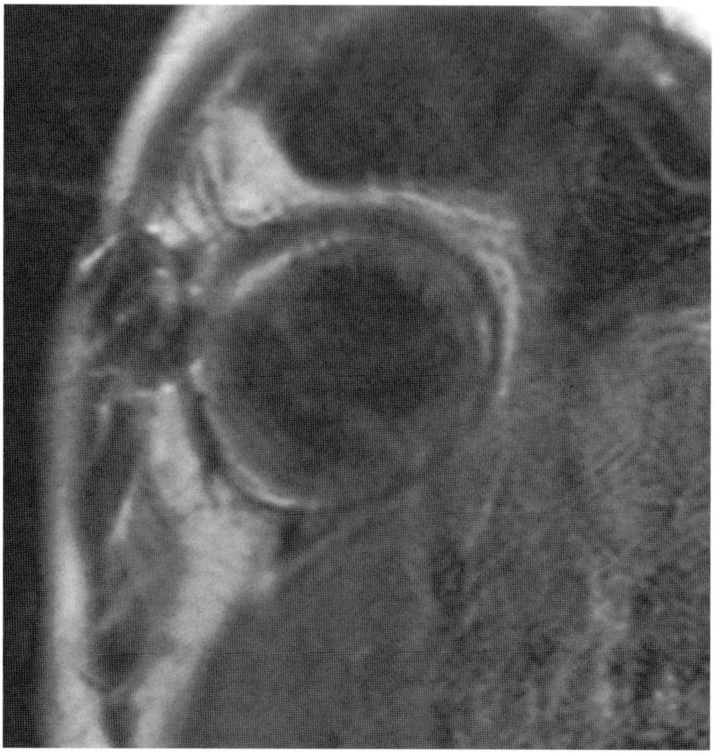

What is the likely diagnosis?

A. Hypertrophic cardiomyopathy
B. Restrictive cardiomyopathy
C. Constrictive pericarditis
D. Right ventricular dysplasia
E. Ischemic cardiomyopathy

Correct answer is C.

The pericardium is normally a thin black line around the heart [1–4]. In this patient, the pericardial is several millimeters thick (> 4 mm) and almost equal to the left ventricular wall thickness. The left ventricular walls are not thinned out and the cavity size is normal, arguing against ischemic cardiomyopathy. In Fig. 4.2, there is also no evidence of restrictive cardiomyopathy (although restrictive cardiomyopathy could certainly not be excluded on the basis of the appearance of the myocardium alone). Finally, there is no evidence of fatty infiltration of the right ventricle. The bright rim around the heart (*asterisks*) is normal epicardial fat.

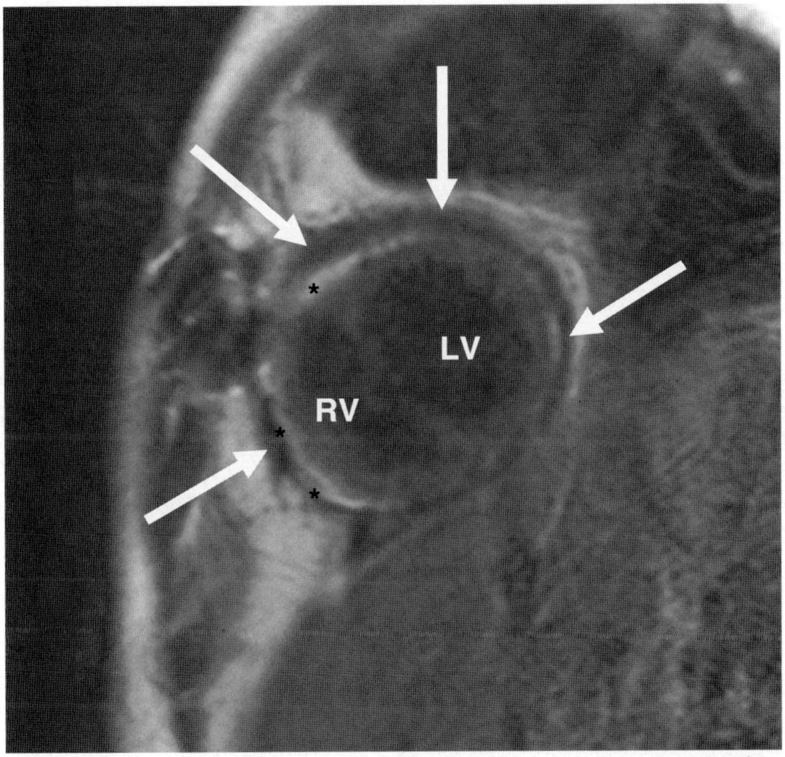

2. A 23-year-old man presents with fever, pleuritic chest pain, diffuse ST segment elevation, and serum troponin level elevation. A clinical diagnosis of viral myocarditis is made.

Which of the following CMR findings would be most consistent with the diagnosis?

A. A dilated and paper-thin right ventricular free wall with areas of fatty infiltration
B. A dilated left ventricle with severe aortic regurgitation
C. A thickened pericardium with normal left ventricular function and no pericardial effusion
D. A normal size left ventricle with focal mid and subepicardial gadolinium enhancement
E. A normal size left ventricle with focal subendocardial gadolinium enhancement

Correct answer is D.

Myocarditis is characterized by diffuse or focal myocardial inflammation that occurs in noncoronary distributions. Typically, mid-wall or subepicardial signal enhancement is seen after gadolinium administration [5–11]. The early enhancement is likely caused by increased blood flow in the area of inflammation, whereas the delayed enhancement may be caused by local expansion of the extracellular space. Endocardial late gadolinium enhancement is typical for nontransmural myocardial infarctions caused by coronary artery disease, spasm, etc. Although viral myocarditis may also affect the right ventricle, the findings are not similar to right ventricular dysplasia. Severe aortic regurgitation can cause left ventricular dilation, but this valvular abnormality is uncommon as a complication of myocarditis. Pericardial thickening is not a finding in acute viral myocarditis.

3. Figure 4.3 is a single slice from a 4-chamber cine loop, obtained during breath holding.

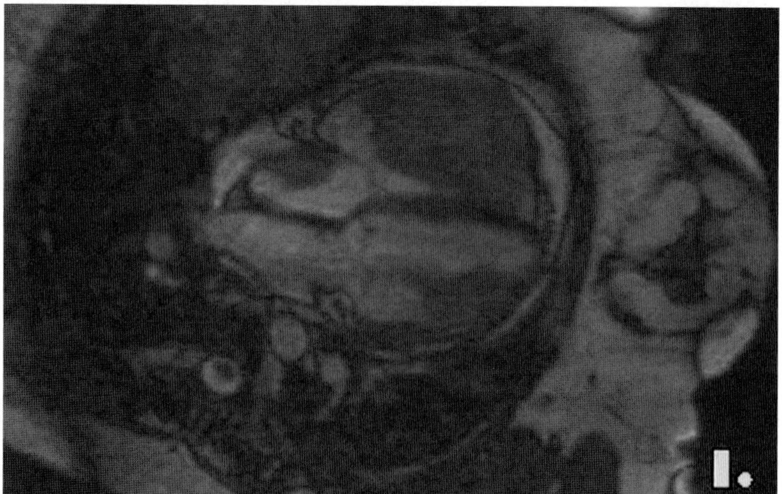

What is the likely diagnosis?

A. Tuberous sclerosis
B. Metastatic malignancy
C. Hypertrophic cardiomyopathy
D. Endomyocardial fibroelastosis
E. Chagas disease

Correct answer is B.

This unfortunate patient has multiple lesions involving the right atrium, right ventricle, and papillary muscle of the left ventricle (Fig. 4.4, *black asterisks*). These lesions distort the normal myocardial anatomy and the lesion involving the right ventricle obliterates most of its cavity. This is undoubtedly metastatic malignancy (in this case, metastatic sarcoma). A pericardial effusion is also evident as a bright rim around the apex of the heart and adjacent to the right atrium (*arrows*). CMR has significant value for assessment of primary and metastatic cardiac masses [12]. Although hypertrophic cardiomyopathy can rarely involve both left and right ventricles [13], involvement of the atrial wall would not be expected.

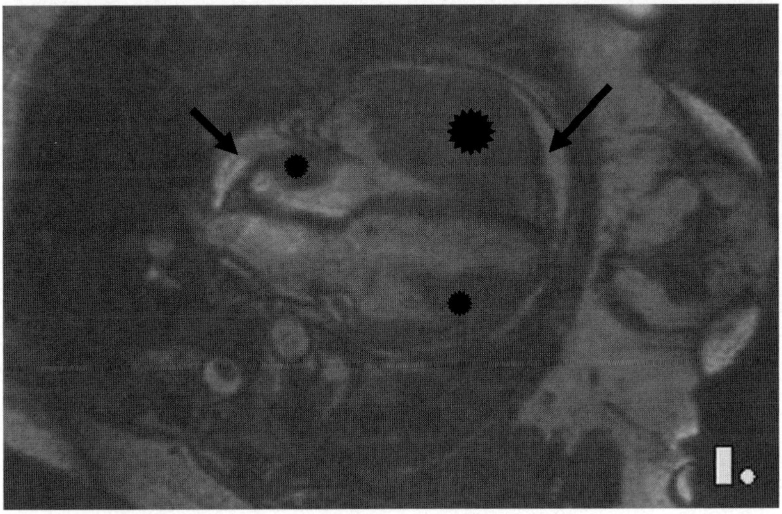

4. Figure 4.5 is a fat-suppressed T2-weighted transverse slice at the level of the coronary sinus in a young man who was incidentally noted to have an abnormal chest X-ray.

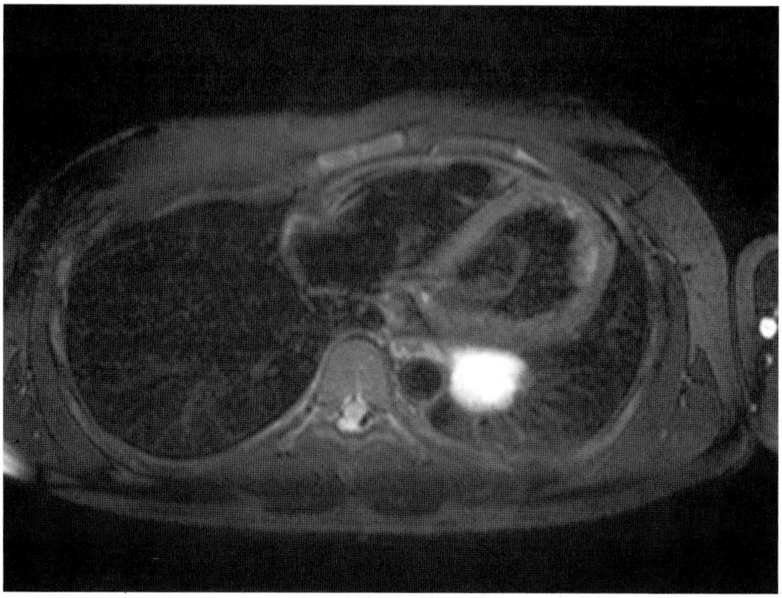

The likely diagnosis is:

A. Hiatal hernia
B. Lipoma
C. Metastatic tumor
D. Pericardial cyst
E. Aortic rupture

Correct answer is D.

Pericardial cysts (*PC*) have high signals in T2-weighted sequences and smooth borders [14, 15]. A lipoma is not suggested, because the sequence is fat-suppressed (note the low signal from the subcutaneous fat in Fig. 4.6). Hiatal hernia can also be excluded, because the esophagus is clearly seen (Fig. 4.6, *arrows*) anterior to the aorta. The high signal intensity of the pericardial cyst fluid cannot be confused with the intermediate signal of a solid mass.

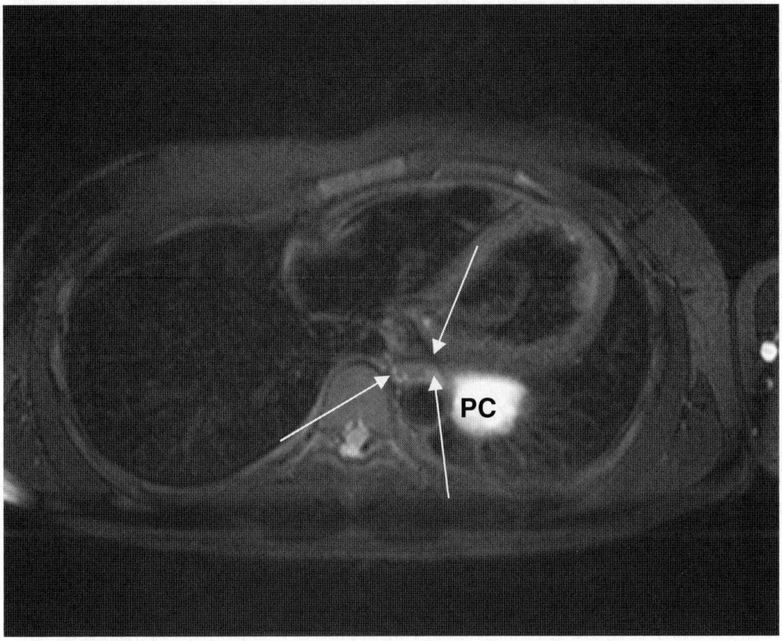

5. The images in Fig. 4.7 are obtained from a real-time (non-ECG-gated) CMR and represent early diastolic images at different parts of the respiratory cycle, during (A) deep inspiration and (B) expiration.

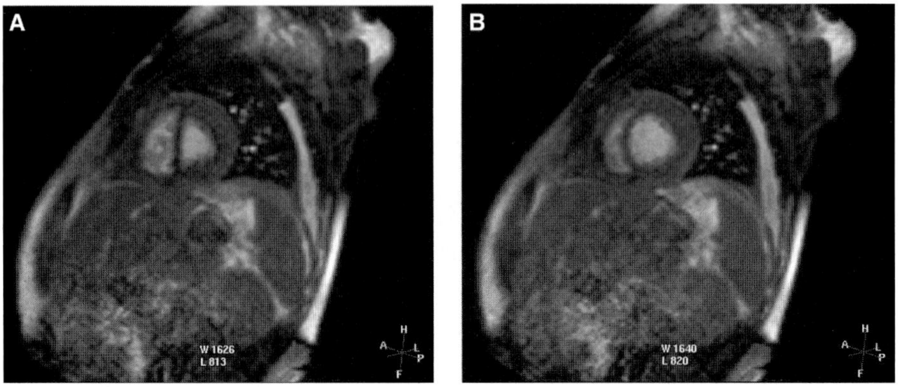

Which is the most likely diagnosis?

A. Hypertrophic cardiomyopathy
B. Ischemic cardiomyopathy
C. Nonischemic cardiomyopathy
D. Constrictive pericarditis
E. Arrhythmogenic right ventricular dysplasia

Correct answer is D.

The images demonstrate an inspiratory increase of the right ventricular size with leftward displacement of the intraventricular septum. During inspiration, the systemic venous return increases because of negative intrathoracic pressure. When the pericardial cavity is noncompliant (e.g., caused by thickening of the pericardium), the right heart pressures rise early at inspiration, resulting in the septal flattening and leftward displacement hereby presented [16, 17]. The apparent asymmetric left ventricular hypertrophy is due to the pericardial thickening adjacent to the lateral left ventricular wall.

6. **A young woman is found to have an intracardiac mass in an echocardiogram performed for mild hypertension. A CMR examination is requested. The transverse images in Fig. 4.8 are obtained. A is a T1-weighted image; B is a T1 weighted image with contrast enhancement; C is a T1-weighted image with suppression of the signal from the adipose tissue; and D is a T2-weighted image.**

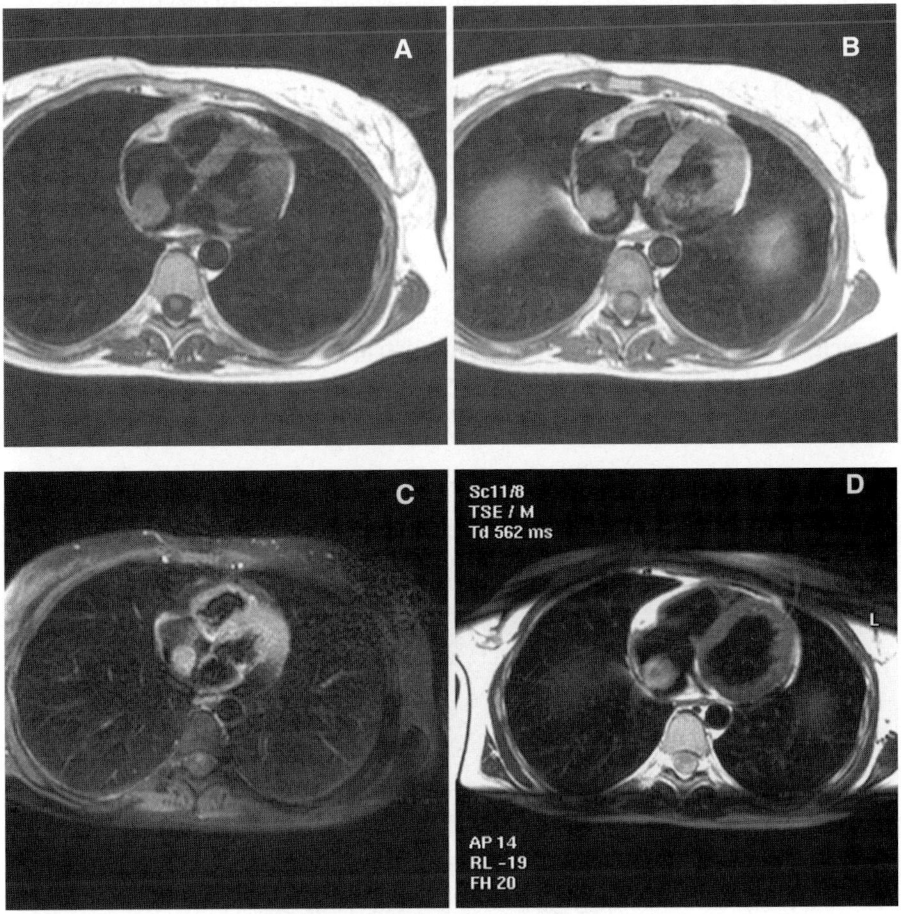

Which is the most likely diagnosis?

A. Thrombus
B. Teratoma
C. Hydatid cyst
D. Myxoma
E. Lipoma

Correct answer is D.

Myxomas are the most common cardiac tumors. They are typically round, well circumscribed, and can have some inhomogeneity of their signal, of their signal both at baseline and after contrast administration. Myxomas are frequently sessile, as this tumor seems to be. The most common location of myxomas is the left atrium, although right atrial myxomas are not uncommon [18–20]. In this case, thrombus is an unlikely diagnosis because of contrast enhancement. Lipoma is also unlikely, because the tumor is still present after fat signal suppression. Hydatid cysts would be very bright in T2-weighted sequences, dark in T1-weighted sequences, and would not take up contrast [21, 22]. Finally, teratomas of the heart are extremely rare, and the consistency (i.e. signal intensity) would be expected to be more inhomogeneous [23].

7. **The images in Fig. 4.9 were obtained in an elderly woman with history of lung cancer who had undergone left pneumonectomy and systemic chemotherapy via a Hickman catheter. A is a proton-density image; B is a T1-weighted image after contrast administration; and C is a T2-weighted image. All images are in the transverse orientation. The thoracic anatomy is severely distorted after removal of the left lung.**

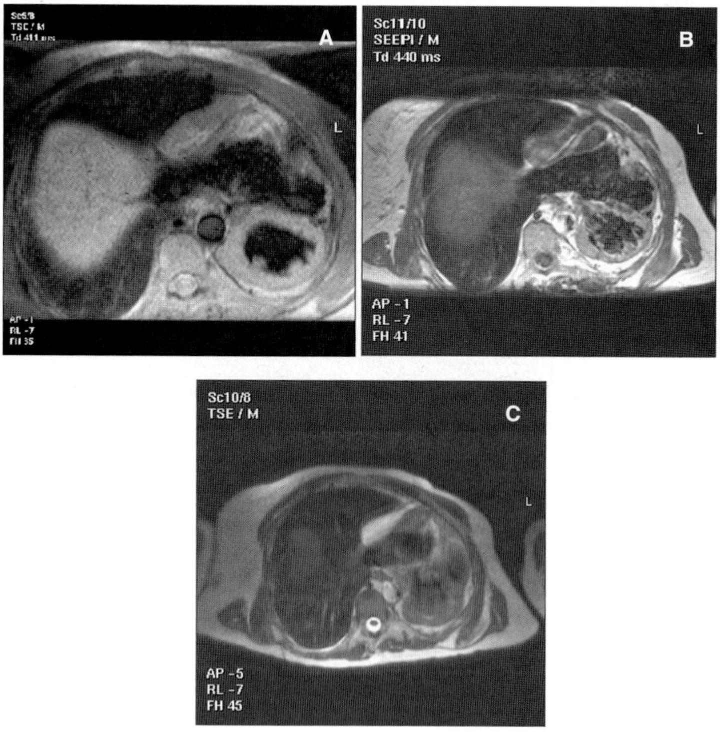

What statement best describes the findings from this study?

A. There is a large hiatal hernia present
B. There is a right lung tumor compressing the right atrium
C. There is a large intracardiac mass, most likely metastatic lung tumor
D. There is bacterial endocarditis of the tricuspid valve with septic pulmonary emboli
E. There is a loculated right pleural effusion and a right atrial mass, most likely thrombus

Correct answer is E.

The loculated right pleural effusion (*Pl. eff*) has high signal in the T2-weighted image (Fig. 4.10C) and does not enhance in the T1-weighted image after contrast administration (Fig. 4.10B). The right atrial mass (*white arrows*) has an intermediate signal in the proton-density images and a low signal in the T2-weighted image. Most importantly, it does not take up contrast at all (Fig. 4.10B), suggesting that the most likely diagnosis is a right atrial clot, possibly related to the Hickman catheter. The esophagus is a posterior mediastinal structure, located far away from the pathology noted in the anterior chest. There is no primary lung parenchymal pathology noted in the right lung in this image.

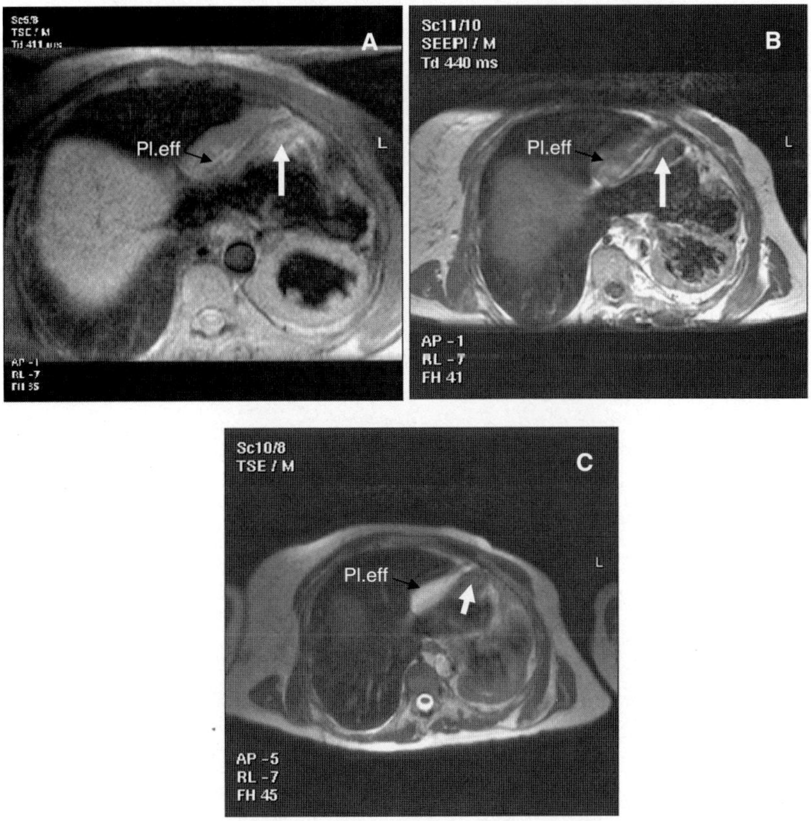

8. Figure 4.11 is a single frame from a cine 4-chamber study obtained from a young obese male with a history of endocarditis.

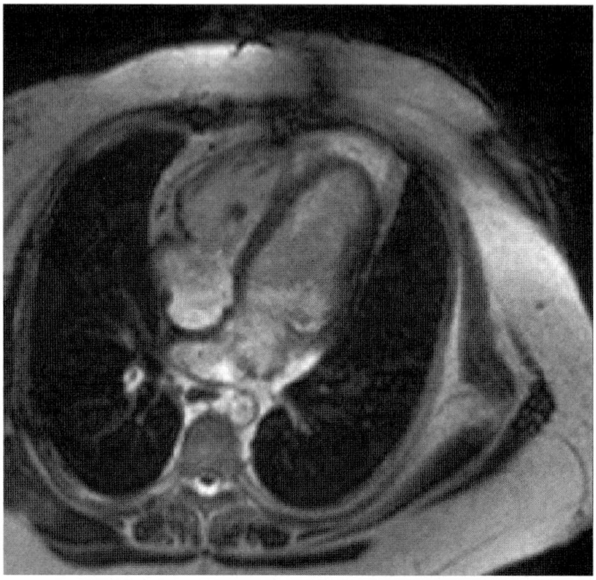

The main finding in this image is:

A. Right atrial mass, possibly vegetation
B. Mitral valve vegetation
C. Pericardial effusion
D. Flow jet from a ventricular septal defect
E. Thickening, possibly vegetation of the tricuspid valve subvalvular apparatus

Correct answer is E.

The *black arrows* in Fig. 4.12 demonstrate thickening, possibly vegetation of the tricuspid valve subvalvular apparatus. CMR is not the most appropriate imaging modality to study small and highly mobile structures (such as vegetations). However, in patients with large vegetations, CMR may be able to demonstrate the pathology. The *white arrow* demonstrates a prominent crista terminalis, which is frequently misinterpreted as a right atrial mass. There is no evidence for mitral valve pathology or ventricular septal defect flow jet. There is no significant pericardial effusion; there is a prominent pericardial fat pad and significant body obesity.

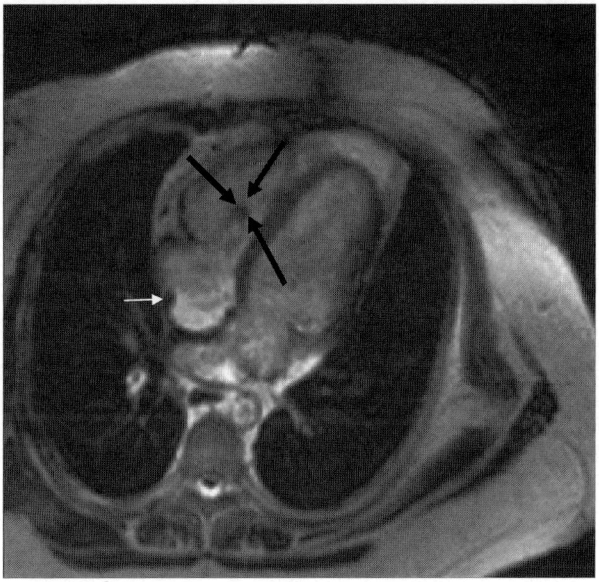

9. The images in Fig. 4.13 are diastolic (A) and systolic (B) frames from a cine short axis study of a young asymptomatic man with family history of sudden cardiac death.

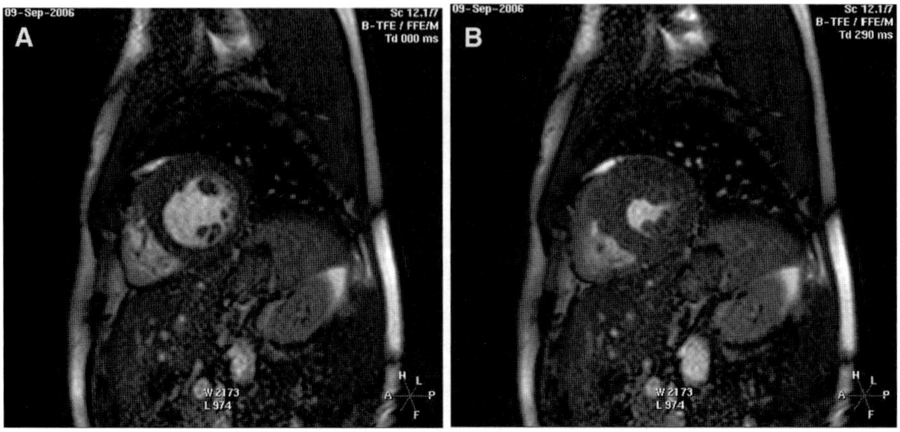

What is the most likely diagnosis?

A. Hypertrophic cardiomyopathy with asymmetric septal hypertrophy
B. Hypertrophic cardiomyopathy, Yamaguchi type
C. Takotsubo cardiomyopathy
D. Noncompaction left ventricle
E. Arrhythmogenic right ventricular dysplasia

Correct answer is A.

The *arrows* on the diastolic frame (Fig. 4.14A) demonstrate significant hypertrophy of the anterior septum and anterior wall, consistent with the diagnosis of hypertrophic cardiomyopathy. The systolic frame (Fig. 4.14B) demonstrates very good systolic function of both left and right ventricles. CMR compares favorably to echocardiography in defining the location and extent of cardiac hypertrophy and providing an accurate measurement of left ventricular mass [24]. The apex is not visualized in these images to suggest either the Yamaguchi type cardiomyoapthy (apical hypertrophic cardiomyopathy) or the Takotsubo cardiomyopathy (apical ballooning, usually induced by acute stress). There is also no evidence for noncompaction cardiomyopathy or arrhythmogenic right ventricular dysplasia.

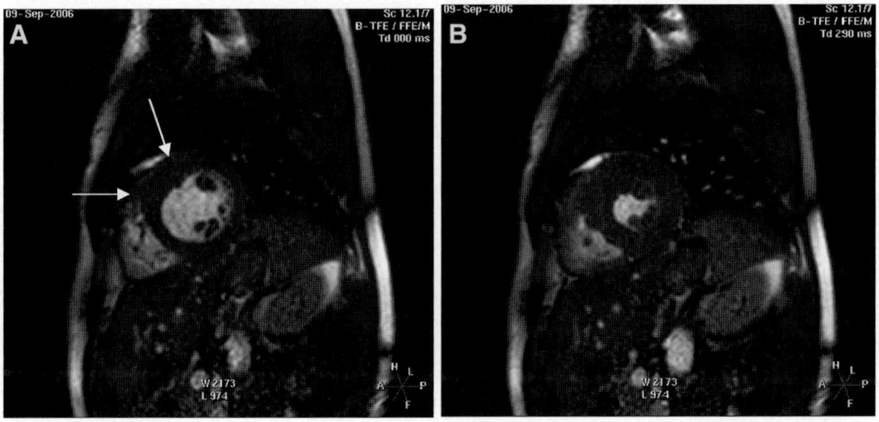

10. The images in Fig. 4.15 were obtained from a young man with shortness of breath. A is a diastolic short axis image; B is a systolic short axis image; C is a diastolic 4-chamber image; and D is a systolic 4-chamber image.

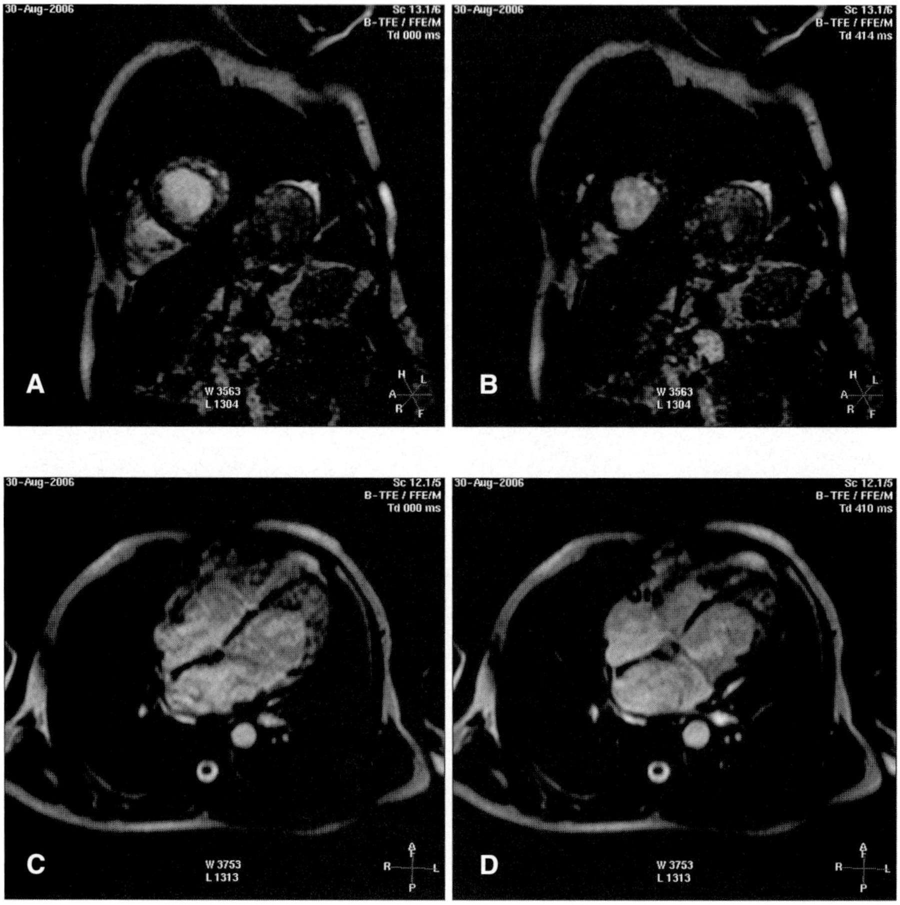

What is the likely diagnosis?

A. Hypertrophic cardiomyopathy with asymmetric septal hypertrophy
B. Apical hypertrophic cardiomyopathy (Yamaguchi)
C. Takotsubo cardiomyopathy
D. Noncompaction cardiomyopathy
E. Arrhythmogenic right ventricular dysplasia

Correct answer is D.

Figure 4.15 demonstrates the typical findings of noncompaction cardiomyoapthy, which are a distinct endocardial layer, separated from the epicardium, usually at the lateral and apical left ventricular walls [25]. The systolic function of the left ventricle is decreased. The right ventricle may also have prominent trabeculations, as is the case in the images shown. There is no evidence for apical or septal hypertrophy, apical ballooning (Takotsubo cardiomyopathy), or isolated arrhythmogenic right ventricular dysplasia.

11. **A 26-year-old woman undergoes CMR as part of a work-up for palpitations. A 4-cm diameter structure is identified anterior to the right atrioventricular groove, extending from the epicardial aspect of the heart to the inner thoracic wall. This structure has smooth contour, low signal in the T1-weighted sequences, and high signal in the T2-weighted sequences. A gadolinium-enhanced T1-weighted sequence does not demonstrate signal enhancement inside the structure, and the delayed images demonstrate no delayed enhancement. The size and function of both right and left ventricles are entirely normal and not affected by the previously described structure. Flow studies of the proximal aorta and pulmonary arteries demonstrate normal flow patterns, with Qp equal to Qs. It is calculated that there is no atrioventricular valve insufficiency. What is the most appropriate next step for the management of this patient?**

    A. Referral to a cardiothoracic surgeon for excision of the identified structure
    B. Needle biopsy of the identified structure
    C. Whole body positron emission tomography for evaluation of possible metastatic disease
    D. Reassurance and follow-up imaging in a few months time
    E. Computed tomography (CT) scan of the chest for evaluation of calcifications related to the identified structure

Correct answer is D.

The patient hereby described has a pericardial cyst. The imaging characteristics (low signal in the T1-weighted sequence, high signal in the T2-weighted sequence, and no early or late gadolinium enhancement) are fairly typical for a cystic structure. The location, size, and smooth contours are also typical for a pericardial cyst [14]. Pericardial cysts are benign and usually do not interfere with cardiac anatomy and function. In these cases, such as the one described here, no specific therapy is required. Drainage of the cyst or surgical excision are rarely indicated, if there is rapid expansion of the cyst or compression of adjacent structures. This patient's palpitations are most likely not related to this incidental finding and, thus, no further diagnostic or therapeutic procedure would be indicated.

12. Which of the following findings is suggestive of poor outcome in an adult patient with thalassemia major?

A. Increase of the myocardial T1 at rest
B. Increase of the myocardial T1 with vasodilation
C. Decrease of the T2* of the myocardium at rest
D. Increase of the T2* of the myocardium at rest
E. Increase of the T2 of the myocardium at rest

Correct answer is C.

Patients with thalassemia major require frequent blood transfusions and are subject to hemochromatosis. Iron deposition in the myocardium is associated with poor outcome. At CMR, myocardial iron deposition results in an decrease of the myocardial T2* (and T2) times [26], which is visually seen as decreased signal in the T2-weighted sequences. T2* can be calculated from a T2 map that is extracted from images of the heart obtained with different echo times (TE) [27, 28]. Severe myocardial iron overload is suggested when the T2* is less than 10 ms [26]. The appearance of the myocardium at rest or after vasodilation at the T1-weighted sequences does not significantly change.

13. In a patient with suspected arrhythmogenic right ventricular dysplasia, all of the following sequences would be helpful in a CMR study *except* for:

A. ECG-gated cine sequence
B. Real-time sequence
C. Fat-suppressed T1-weighted black blood sequence
D. T1-weighted black blood sequence
E. Time-of-flight sequence

Correct answer is E.

ECG-gated cine sequences are the mainstay for evaluation of left and right ventricular function. Real-time sequences can be used to assess ventricular function in patients with significant arrhythmia that hinders ECG-gated acquisitions. T1- and T2-weighted anatomic imaging with black blood sequences can nicely demonstrate fatty infiltration in patients with arrhythmogenic right ventricular dysplasia, as islets of bright tissue (fat) inside the myocardium (grey). Fat-suppressed imaging is also of value to confirm that the bright signal is indeed from adipose tissue (which now should become dark), and not artifactual. Time-of-flight is a sequence used for MR angiography, which would not be of value in evaluation of possible arrhythmogenic right ventricular dysplasia.

14. Figure 4.16 shows diastolic (A) and systolic (B) images from a cine CMR study obtained at the 4-chamber orientation with a technique called spatial modulation of magnetization (SPAMM) tagging.

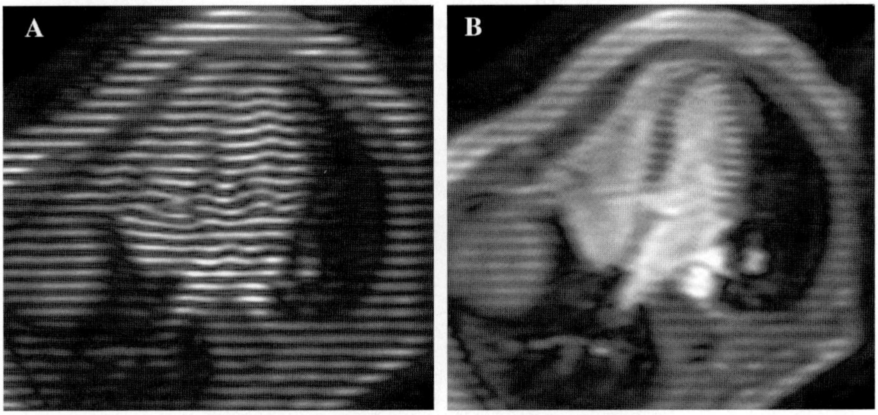

Which of the following pathologic conditions/diseases would *not* be addressed with this technique?

A. Arrhythmogenic right ventricular dysplasia
B. Constrictive pericarditis
C. Assessment of myocardial viability
D. Mitral valve prolapse with significant regurgitation
E. Myocarditis

Correct answer is D.

SPAMM and other myocardium tagging techniques allow the assessment of regional myocardial contraction and rotation/counter-rotation [29]. Thus, the greatest value of this technique is for evaluation of diseases that may be associated with a focal or global wall motion abnormality (coronary artery disease, myocarditis, and cardiomyopathies). This technique can also assess the epicardial motion in relation to the pericardium and surrounding tissues, which can be of value for diagnosis of constrictive pericarditis. In patients with pericardial constriction, the epicardium is adherent to the thickened and/or inflamed pericardium and cannot perform the normal base to apex sliding motion. Myocardial tagging has no value for assessment of valvular disease; the technique to quantify blood flow is called phase contrast (or velocity encoding).

15. A young nulliparous female patient presented to the emergency department with fever and chest pain. Initial laboratory evaluation showed an increased plasma troponin level. An echocardiogram showed decreased left ventricular systolic function. A CMR was performed that confirmed the mild left ventricular systolic dysfunction. The delayed contrast-enhanced 4-chamber image is shown in Fig. 4.17.

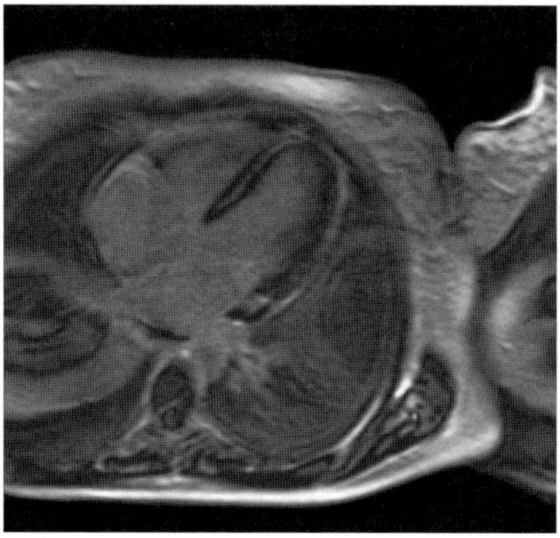

The most likely diagnosis is:

A. Viral myocarditis
B. Libman–Sachs endocarditis
C. Myocardial infarction caused by coronary artery disease
D. Myocardial infarction caused by cocaine abuse
E. Pregnancy-related cardiomyopathy

Correct answer is A.

The delayed contrast-enhanced 4-chamber image demonstrates mid-wall enhancement, particularly at the intraventricular septum (Fig. 4.18, *white arrows*).

This finding is characteristic of acute myocarditis and nonischemic cardiomyopathy [5, 11]. In contrast, the myocardial infarction pattern involves endocardial signal enhancement at the delayed contrast-enhanced images with variable transmural extension, because the endocardium is always the first myocardial layer to be affected by ischemia. This pattern is irrespective of the cause of decreased blood flow (acute coronary thrombosis caused by atherosclerotic coronary disease, vessel spasm caused by cocaine, etc.). Although lupus carditis might be considered in the differential diagnosis in the appropriate context, Libman–Sachs endocarditis does not typically have myocardial involvement. Finally, the CMR image might be con-

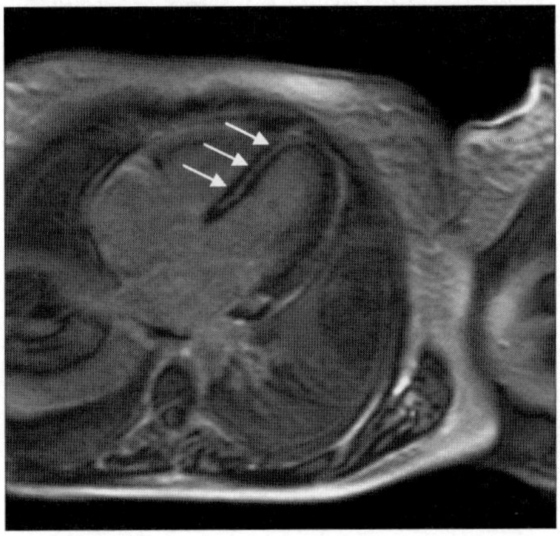

sistent with pregnancy-related cardiomyopathy, but the clinical presentation is not suggestive of this diagnosis. Pregnancy-related cardiomyopathy occurs typically peripartum and is not associated with fever and signs of acute inflammation.

A word of caution: an artifactual mid-wall enhancement may be the result of an incorrect selection of the inversion time for the contrast-enhanced images. One should always evaluate more than a single inversion time to assure adequate myocardial signal nulling. In this patient, nulling of the entire myocardium could not be achieved at several different inversion times. The diagnosis was also supported from the early T1-weighted images that demonstrated early mid-wall enhancement, a finding suggestive of active inflammation (Fig. 4.19).

In Fig. 4.19, the *left panel* is a T1-weighted transverse image before contrast administration. The *right panel* is a T1-weighted image at the same location shortly after the administration of intravenous 0.2 mmol/kg gadolinium. The *arrows* demonstrate mid-wall enhancement at the intraventricular septum, a finding suggestive of active inflammation.

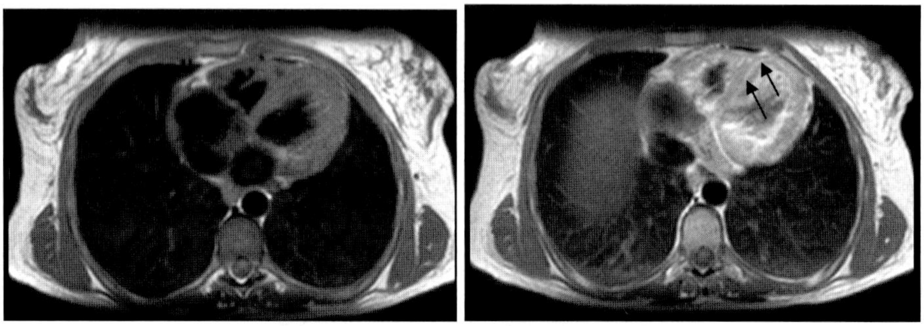

16. The T1-weighted images in Fig. 4.20 were obtained from a young man with dyspnea, before (A) and after (B) administration of paramagnetic contrast agent (gadolinium).

What is the likely diagnosis?

A. Cardiac tumor
B. Pulmonary embolism
C. Atrial septal defect
D. Arrhythmogenic right ventricular dysplasia
E. Constrictive pericarditis

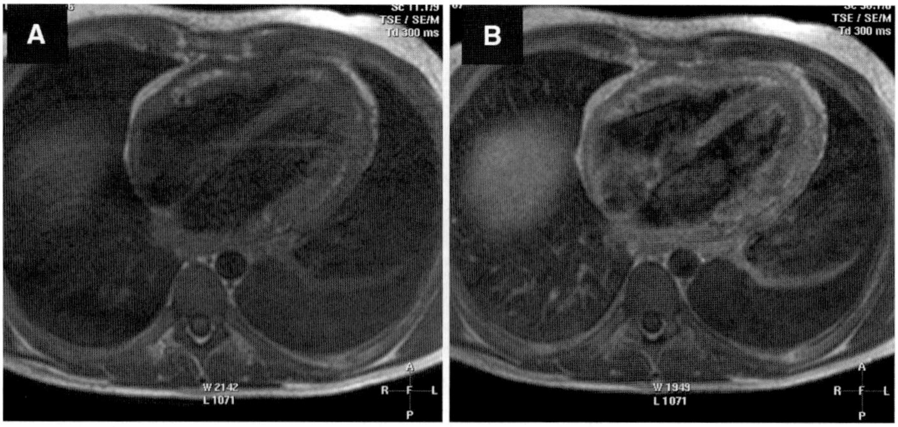

Correct answer is E.

The images in Fig. 4.21 demonstrate the following abnormal findings:

i. Circumferentially thickened pericardium (dark rim around the heart indicated by *white arrows*)
ii. Pericardial contrast uptake (*white arrowheads*)
iii. Left pleural effusion (*asterisk*)

These findings are suggestive of constrictive pericarditis with active inflammation. The pericardium is considered thickened when it is >4 mm [2, 3, 14, 15]. In this case, the thickness of the pericardium adjacent to the left ventricular wall was 10 mm. The pericardial contrast uptake suggests increased blood flow consistent with active inflammation. The right heart size is normal, arguing against intracardiac shunt, arrhythmogenic right ventricle, or pulmonary embolism. There is no evidence of cardiac mass.

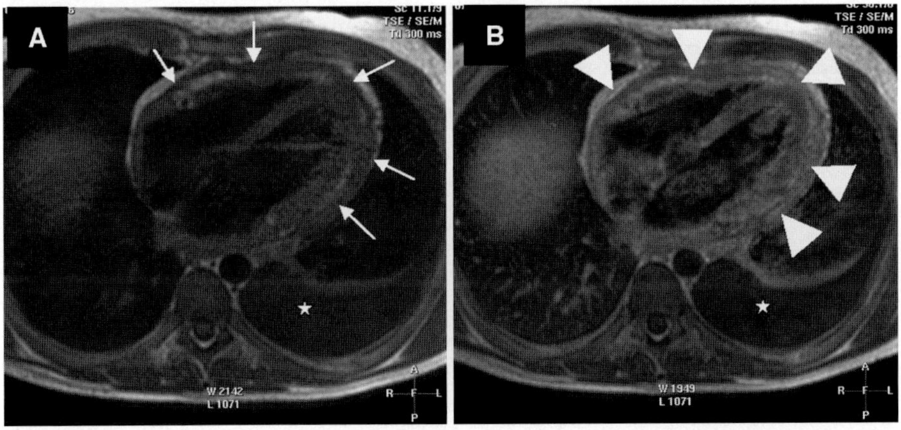

17. The transverse images in Fig. 4.22 were obtained from a 70-year-old woman with dyspnea New York Heart Association (NYHA) class IV. A and B are T1-weighted images before and after contrast, respectively; C is a T2-weighted image; and D is a delayed-enhanced inversion-recovery image. Before the CMR study, transthoracic echocardiography demonstrated pulmonary artery hypertension (>100 mmHg), and chest CT scan showed a filling defect inside the main and the left pulmonary arteries. Which of the following statements best represents the findings from this study?

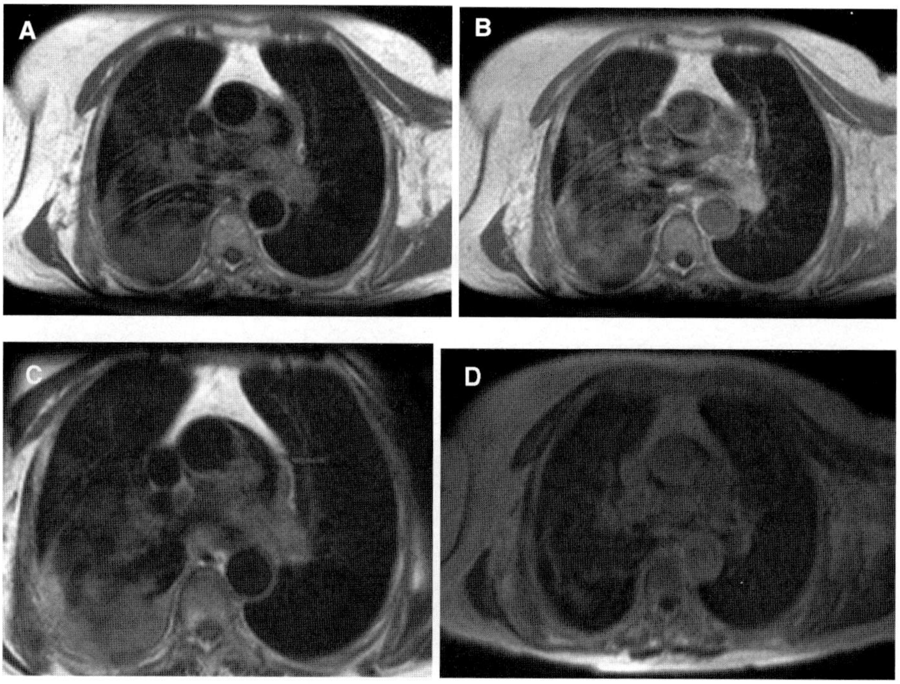

A. The filling defect inside the left pulmonary artery is a clot. A right pleural effusion is also noted, possibly related to pulmonary embolic events in the contralateral side

B. The filling defect inside the left pulmonary artery is a clot. There are no pleural effusions; the abnormal signal noted at the posterior right lung field is likely consolidation from pneumonia/atelectasis

C. The pulmonary artery trunk and left pulmonary artery are compressed from the outside from a large mass involving the ascending aorta and obliterating most of the aortic lumen

D. The pulmonary artery trunk and left pulmonary artery are compressed from the outside from a large mass involving the descending thoracic aorta and obliterating most of the aortic lumen

E. The filling defect inside the left pulmonary artery is a mass (likely malignancy). A right pleural effusion is also noted

Correct answer is E.

The T1-weighted images demonstrate an irregular-shaped structure inside the main and left pulmonary arteries, which obliterates most of the lumen of the left pulmonary artery. After contrast administration, these structures are enhanced (Fig. 4.23B, *arrows*), suggesting increased vascularity. A clot would not take up contrast and, in the delayed-enhanced images, would completely lack signal, similar to what is seen at the right pleural effusion. Although histologic diagnosis cannot be made on the basis of the CMR examination alone, the study suggests malignancy based on the location of the mass and its imaging characteristics. *AAo*, ascending aorta; *DAo*, descending aorta.

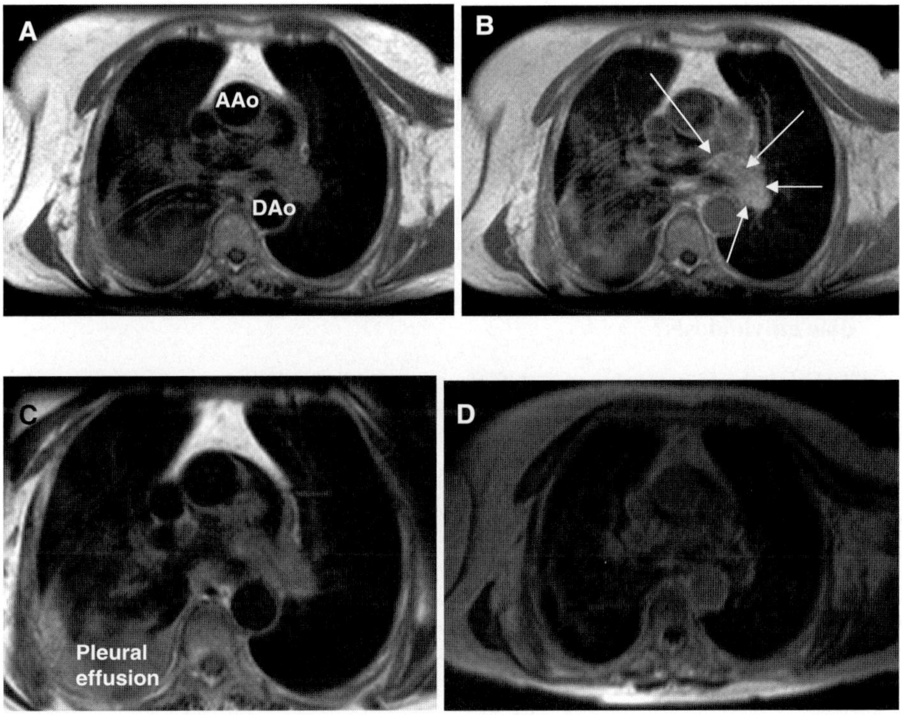

18. In patients with thalassemia major, if there is myocardial iron overload, the myocardium is expected to appear:

A. Brighter than usual
B. Darker than usual
C. Exactly as usual. The effect of myocardial iron overload can only be quantitatively measured
D. Exactly as usual. The effect of myocardial iron overload cannot be measured by conventional MR imaging techniques; spectroscopy, however, can help
E. Sometimes brighter than usual and sometimes darker, depending on the sequence used

Correct answer is B.

Iron is a ferromagnetic ion that inside a magnetic field induces significant susceptibility artifacts, which invariably result in signal loss. Thus, the iron-overloaded myocardium (and for that matter any other organ) will appear darker than usual in CMR. The extent of iron overload can be assessed with conventional CMR sequences by measuring the T2 and T2* times of the myocardium [26].

19. A patient with multiple myeloma and heart failure is referred for a CMR study. Which of the following findings would be most consistent with cardiac amyloidosis?

A. Dilated and hyperdynamic left ventricle with small atria
B. Thickened pericardium
C. Asymmetric septal hypertrophy
D. Patchy myocardial uptake of contrast, with difficult to completely suppress myocardial signal with inversion-recovery sequences obtained 20 minutes after contrast administration
E. Focal subendocardial delayed contrast enhancement with regional wall motion abnormality

Correct answer is D.

The typical appearance of the heart in amyloidosis includes normal size ventricles with normal or concentrically hypertrophied walls and severely dilated atria. The pathophysiology is that of restrictive cardiomyopathy. The deposition of amyloid protein at the interstitium of the myocardium results in expansion of the extracellular space and, thus, increases the volume of distribution for paramagnetic contrast agents (e.g., gadolinium). Therefore, with delayed imaging after contrast administration, the suppression of myocardial signal using inversion-recovery sequences is difficult and usually incomplete, because of the increased gadolinium content of the entire myocardium [30–32]. Patchy uptake can also be seen in cases with more regional involvement. Subendocardial enhancement is more suggestive of coronary artery disease with nontransmural infarction.

20. Which of the following imaging characteristic is *not* suggestive of malignant nature of a cardiac mass?

A. Invasion of the myocardium, pericardium, and extracardiac tissues
B. Inhomogeneous contrast enhancement
C. Presence of hilar lymphadenopathy
D. Presence of a large pericardial effusion
E. Sessile growth with a narrow stalk

Correct answer is E.

Malignant tumors typically have increased vascularity and, thus, demonstrate early contrast enhancement, albeit inhomogeneous [12, 19, 20]. Invasion of other structures is obviously a sign of malignancy, as is the presence of lymphadenopathy and a large pericardial effusion. Sessile cardiac masses with a narrow stalk are usually benign and most commonly are vegetations or myxomas.

21. A middle-age man presents with progressive shortness of breath. The diagnosis of pericardial constriction is entertained based on clinical and echocardiographic data. A CMR study is obtained. Figure 4.24 shows a transverse T1-weighted image (A) and real-time early diastolic frames during expiratory (B) and inspiratory (C) phase of the breathing cycle. The dotted line demonstrates the relative position of the diaphragm at B and C.

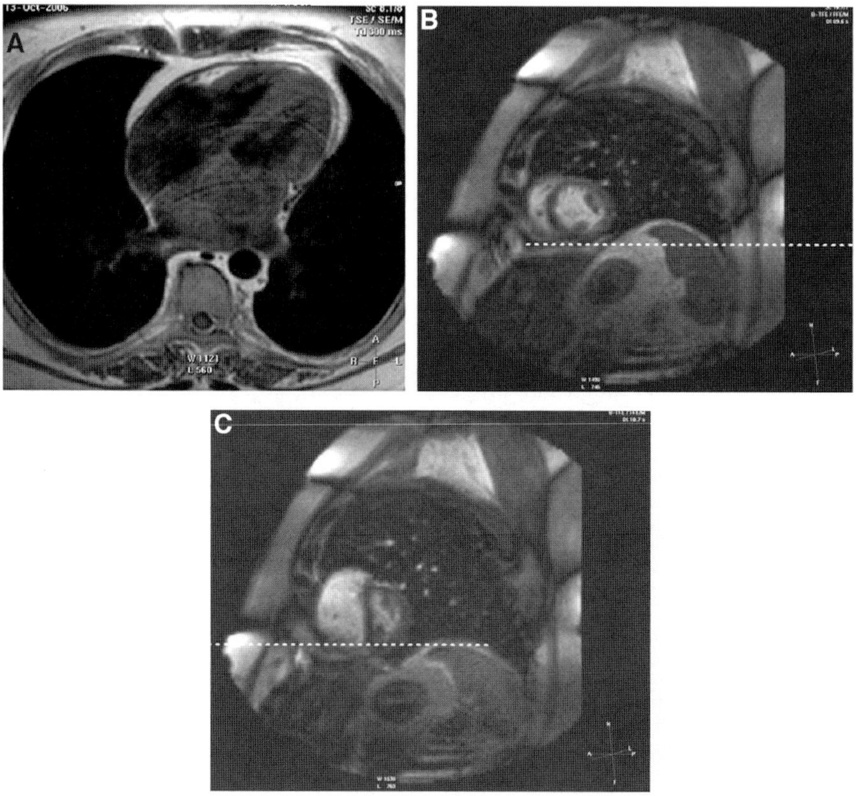

Which of the following statements is most appropriate based on the CMR study?

A. There is pericardial thickening and right ventricular dilation consistent with pericardial constriction
B. There is significant biatrial enlargement and physiologic evidence for restrictive cardiomyopathy
C. There is pericardial effusion with tamponade physiology
D. There is no significant pericardial thickening, but constrictive physiology is evident
E. The patient has primarily lung disease; there is no primary cardiac involvement

Correct answer is D.

The pericardium is considered thickened when it measures >4 mm. In Fig. 4.25A, the pericardium (*opposing arrows*) is <4 mm and comparable in size to the left internal mammary artery (LIMA), shown with a *dotted arrow*. However, the real-time images (*B* and *C*) demonstrate a significant change of the shape of the left ventricle at inspiration. This is because there is a shift of the intraventricular septum toward the left, apparently from transiently increased pressures in the right ventricle. This is consistent with constrictive physiology, where right heart pressures rapidly increase with the increased systemic venous return at inspiration, because the unelastic pericardium cannot accommodate an increase of the total cardiac volume [16, 17].

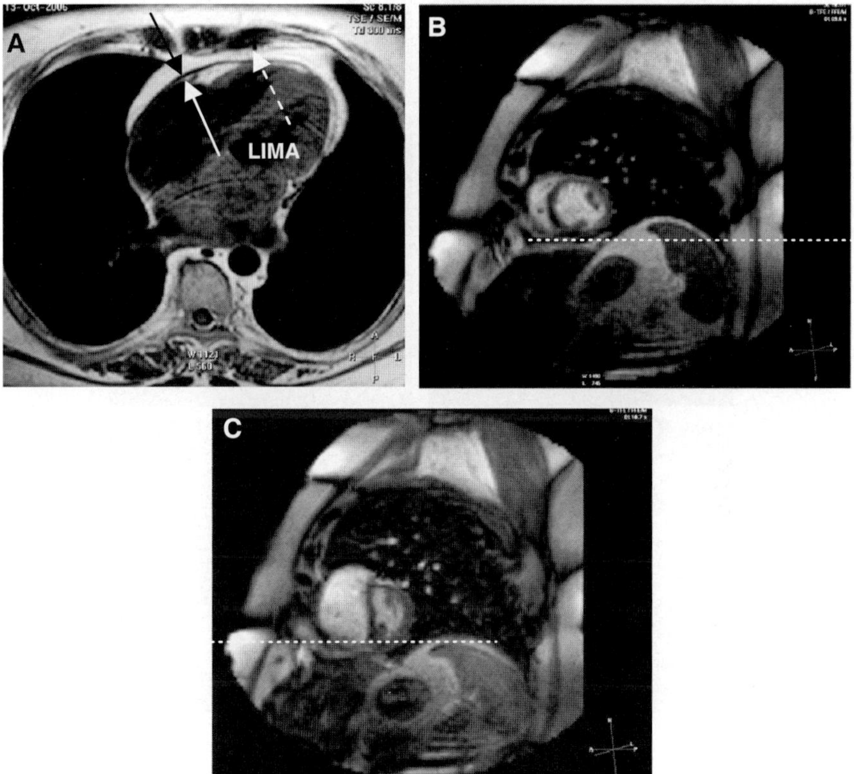

22. A middle-aged man with combined thalassemia major and sickle cell disease is referred for a CMR study for evaluation of shortness of breath. The images in Fig. 4.26 are end-diastolic (left panels) and end-systolic (right panels) frames from the functional cine study in the 2-chamber, 4-chamber, and short-axis orientations.

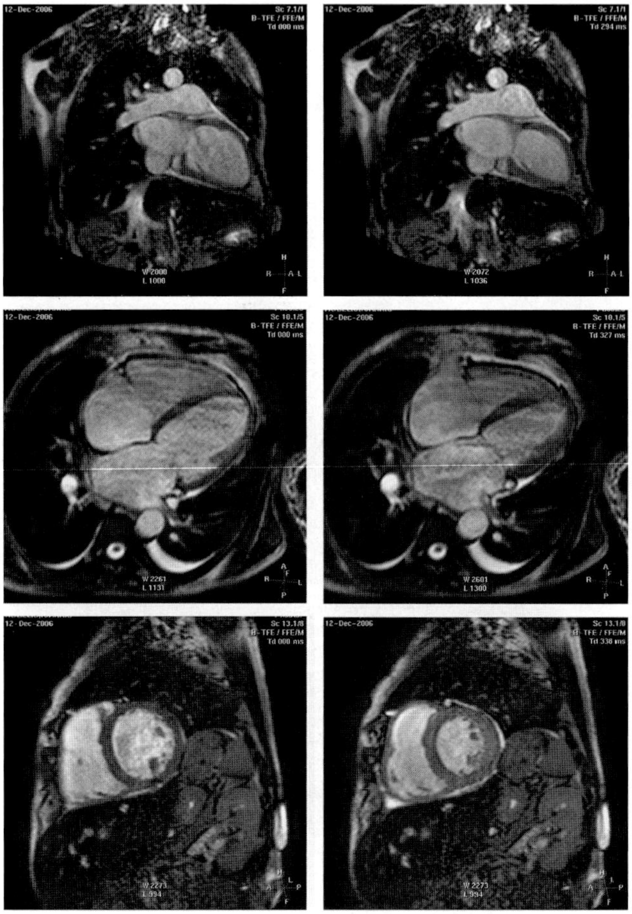

What is the most likely cause of the dyspnea?

A. Severe lobar pneumonia
B. Pulmonary infarcts
C. Pulmonary veno-occlusive disease
D. Epicardial coronary artery disease with previous myocardial infarction(s)
E. Nonischemic cardiomyopathy

Correct answer is E.

The images demonstrate uniform wall thickness, arguing against myocardial infarctions in major epicardial coronary arteries. All walls appear to be moderately hypokinetic. Indeed, using the disk-area method (Simpson's rule) in contiguous short-axis slices, the left ventricular ejection fraction was measured at 41%. There are bilateral small pleural effusions (evident in the 4-chamber slices), corroborating the diagnosis of congestive heart failure as the cause of dyspnea. Chronic anemia with subsequent persistent tachycardia and hyperdynamic circulation could be additional factors contributing to global left ventricular systolic dysfunction. In situ pulmonary thrombosis and veno-occlusive disease are common in patients with sickle cell disease, but their presence could not explain the left-sided heart failure evident in this case. There are no signs of lobar pneumonia on this image.

23. A middle-aged man is referred for a CMR study because at a routine transthoracic echocardiogram a small mass (~1cm) was seen in the right ventricle, attached to the tricuspid valve subvalvular apparatus. The images in Fig. 4.27 (facing page) were obtained. A, transverse T1-weighted image before contrast administration; B, fat-suppressed transverse T1-weighted image before contrast administration; C, transverse T1-weighted image after contrast administration (Gd-DTPA 0.2 mmol/kg); D, diastolic image from an ECG-gated cine study in the 4-chamber orientation; and E, systolic image from an ECG-gated cine study in the 4-chamber orientation.

Which statement best describes the findings from this study?

A. No mass is identified in the cine study. The vaguely defined structure with increased signal in the anatomic images is likely flow-related artifact
B. There is a small mass on the tricuspid valve apparatus and it is most likely a lipoma
C. There is a small mass on the tricuspid valve apparatus and it is most likely an old and calcified vegetation. It is not evident in the cine images because it is highly mobile
D. The referring physician was wrong—the mass is not in the right ventricle but instead on the aortic valve, as is evident from the diastolic 4-chamber cine image
E. There is likely a small, mobile, non-lipomatous and vascular structure on the tricuspid valve subvalvular apparatus

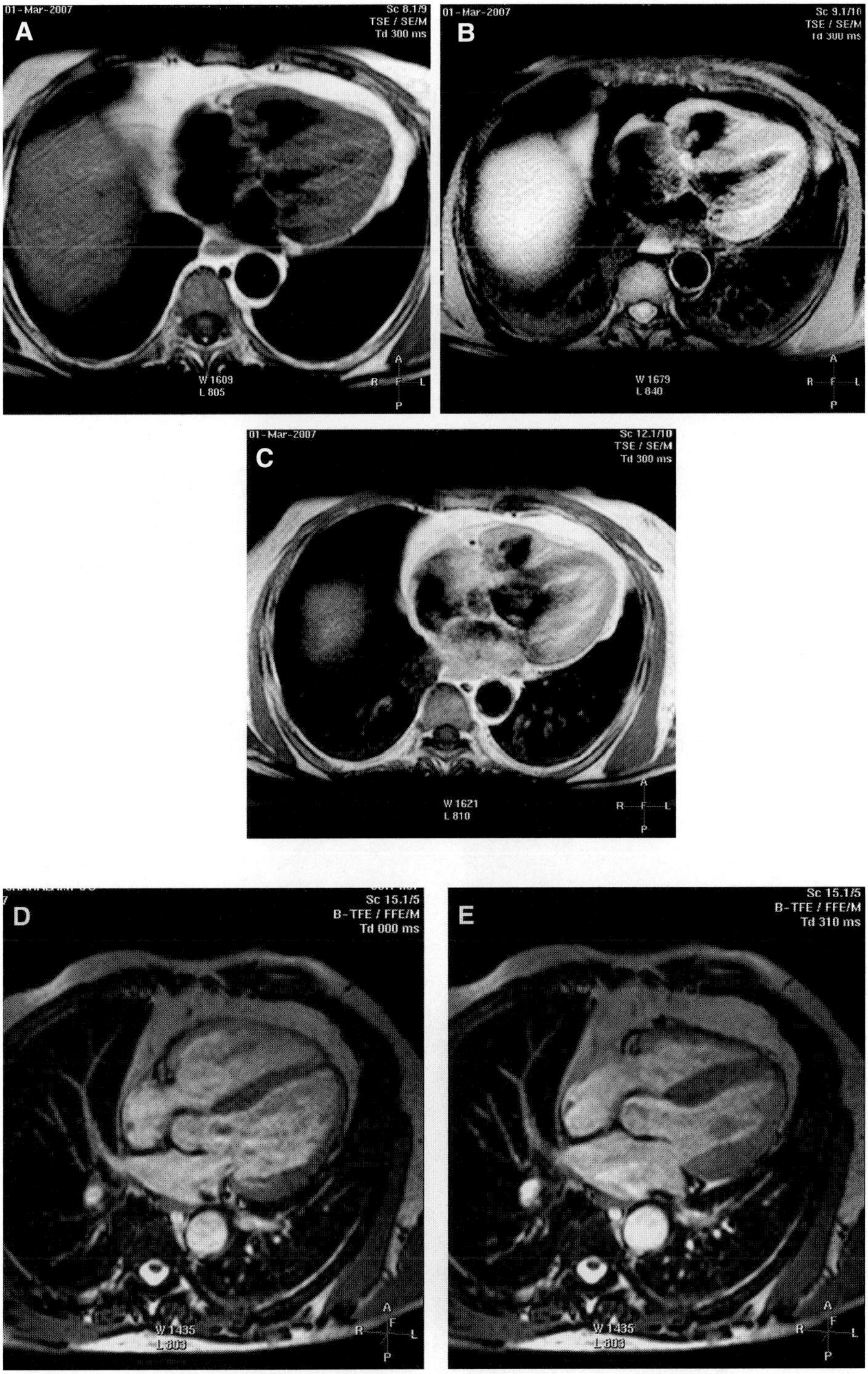
A
01-Mar-2007
Sc 8.1/9
TSE / SE/M
Td 300 ms
W 1609
L 805
B
01-Mar-2007
Sc 9.1/10
TSE / SE/M
W 1679
L 840
C
01-Mar-2007
Sc 12.1/10
TSE / SE/M
Td 300 ms
W 1621
L 810
D
Sc 15.1/5
B-TFE / FFE/M
Td 000 ms
W 1435
E
Sc 15.1/5
B-TFE / FFE/M
Td 310 ms
W 1435

Correct answer is E.

The anatomic images show a vaguely defined structure inside the right ventricle, close to the anterior leaflet of the tricuspid valve (Fig. 4.28, *white arrows*). This structure is still visible after suppression of the signal from adipose tissue (*B*) and, thus, is *not* a lipoma (or other fat containing structure). At the contrast enhanced image (*C*), this structure appears to take up contrast, similar to the surrounding myocardium. Early contrast enhancement argues that this structure is probably vascular and not vegetation. In particular, the presence of calcifications on a vegetation would result in signal loss from susceptibility effects, which makes this diagnosis even less likely. The signal void in the diastolic image of the cine study (*black arrowhead*) is likely due to aortic regurgitation. The right ventricular mass is not seen in the cine study. Highly mobile structures can be missed in an ECG-gated study, where the images are composed from data acquired over several cardiac cycles and the exact location of such a mobile structure could differ from beat to beat.

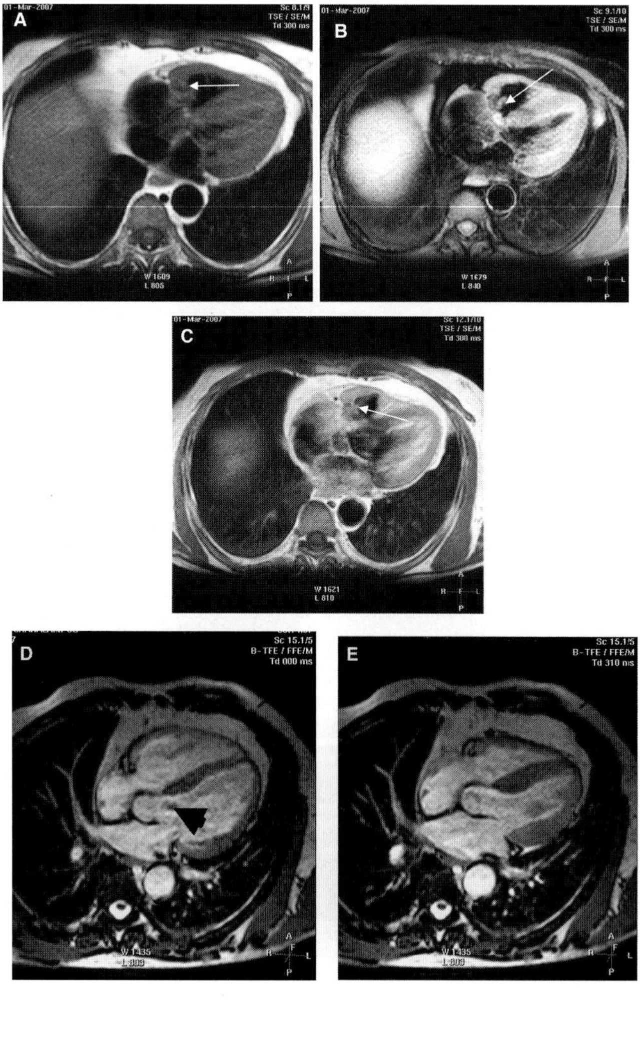

24. In the case described in Question 23, delayed images are also obtained approximately 20 minutes after contrast administration, using an inversion-recovery sequence with heavy T1 weighting. The 4-chamber image is displayed in Fig. 4.29. What is the likely diagnosis?

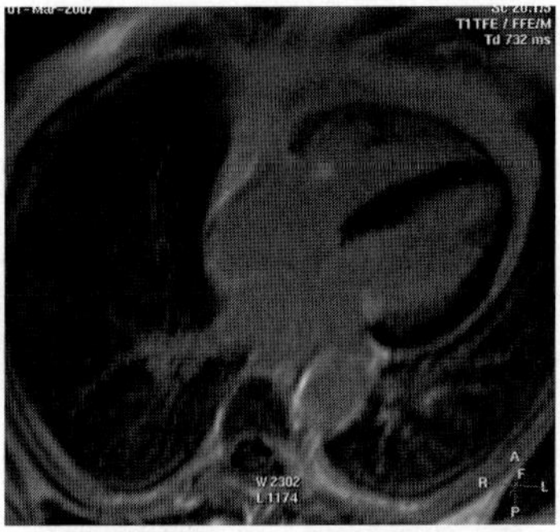

A. Degenerative calcifications
B. Intracardiac thrombi
C. Vegetations
D. Papillary fibroelastomas
E. Slow flow with artifactual flow enhancement below the atrioventricular valves

Correct answer is D.

Figure 4.30 demonstrates two bright small structures, one in the left (*white arrow*) and one in the right ventricle (*black arrow*), both of which appear to be related to the atrioventricular valves. The heavy T1-weighting of this image suggests that bright signal is related to contrast retention. The two identified structures are very discrete and could not be flow-related artifacts. It is also unlikely that these structures are vegetations or thrombi, because neither of these pathologies would take up and retain contrast. Calcifications present as signal voids in all sequences. Thus, the most likely diagnosis is multiple papillary fibroelastomas, a rather uncommon condition [33].

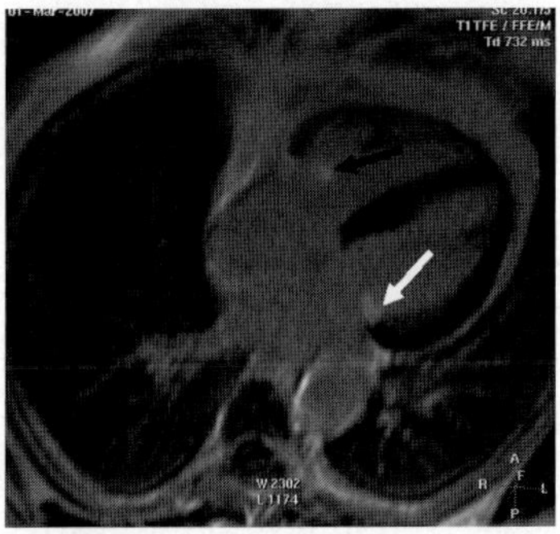

25. A 40-year-old man with an uncertain history of coronary artery disease is referred for a CMR study by an electrophysiologist to "rule out arrhythmogenic right ventricular dysplasia" because of persistent ventricular arrhythmias. The images in Fig. 4.31 are obtained: A and B, diastolic and systolic images, respectively, from a cine study in the 4-chamber orientation; C and D, delayed contrast-enhanced images in the 4-chamber and short-axis orientation, respectively.

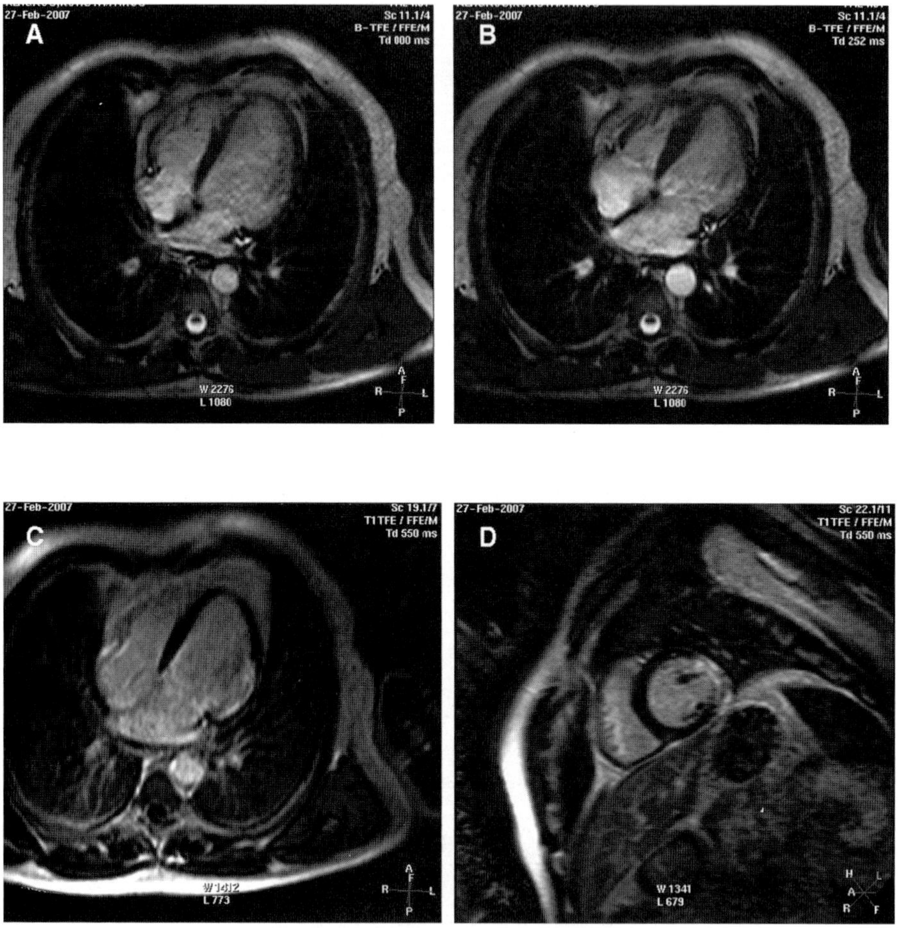

What is the likely diagnosis?

A. Arrhythmogenic right ventricular dysplasia
B. Hemochromatosis
C. Hypertrophic cardiomyopathy
D. Coronary artery disease with infarct in the distribution of the right coronary artery
E. Coronary artery disease with infarct in the distribution of the left circumflex coronary artery

Correct answer is E.

The cine images in Fig. 4.32 demonstrate diastolic thinning of the basal lateral wall (*A, arrows*), with dyskinesis and absence of systolic thickening (*B, arrow*). This area is typically the distribution of the left circumflex coronary artery. The delayed contrast-enhanced viability images demonstrate near transmural hyperenhancement in the same territory (*C* and *D, arrows*), suggesting absence of myocardial viability in the infarct territory [34–36]. Myocardial infarctions in the high lateral wall may be difficult to diagnose, because they are frequently electrocardiographically silent. Indeed, in this patient, electrocardiography failed to establish the diagnosis. The right ventricular size and systolic function are normal and there is no hyperenhancement of the right ventricular free wall, making the diagnosis of arrhythmogenic right ventricular dysplasia unlikely [37, 38]. Hemochromatosis is characterized by iron deposition on the myocardium and usually presents as a nonischemic (dilated) cardiomyopathy. There are no focal areas of hyperenhancement (aka necrosis) associated with hemochromatosis.

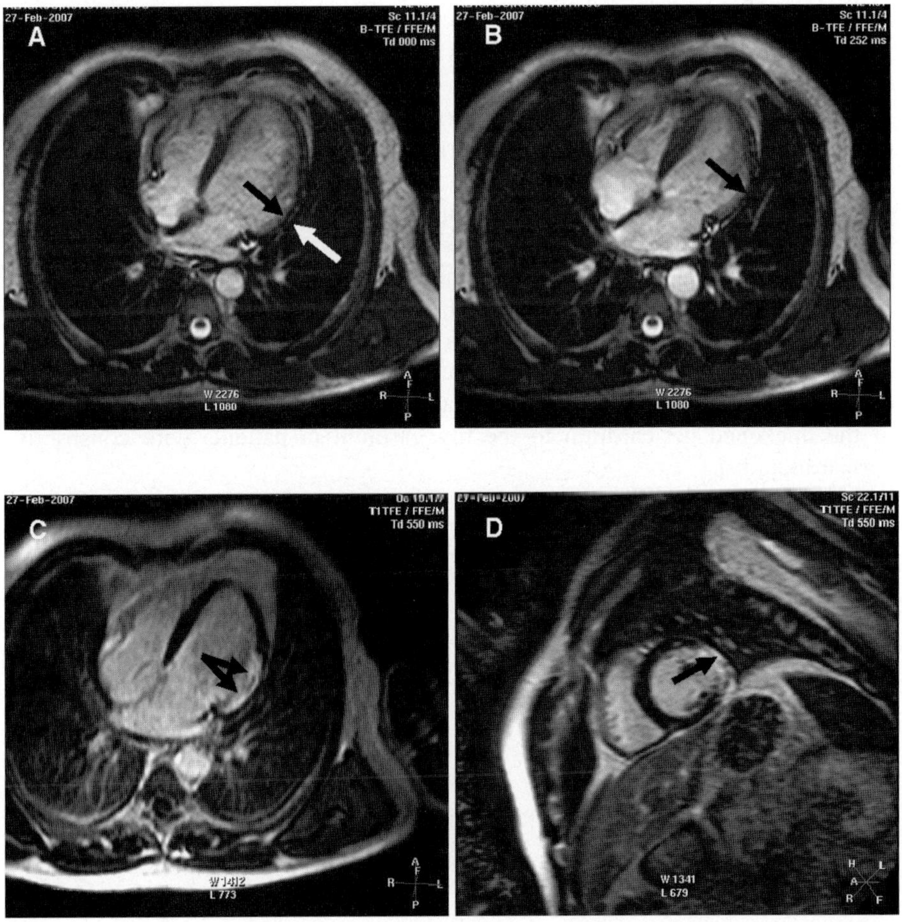

26. A 45-year-old patient is referred for a CMR study for assessment of possible constrictive pericarditis. T1-weighted images in the transverse orientation demonstrate normal pericardial thickness (2 mm). The technologist asks you what should be done next?

A. Stop the study. Refer for a the patient multislice CT scan
B. Perform a cine study using breathholding and a real-time sequence in the 4-chamber orientation
C. Perform a cine study at deep inspiration and expiration using a real-time sequence in the short-axis orientation
D. Perform a cine study at deep inspiration and expiration using a real-time sequence in the 2-chamber (long-axis) orientation
E. Stop the study. No need to take further action. The patient does not have pericardial constriction

Correct answer is C.

Pericardial constriction can indeed occur without pericardial thickening in patients with anelastic pericardium. This is why evaluation of possible pericardial constriction should also include evaluation of the so-called "constrictive physiology." Inspiration is associated with a deep decrease of the intrathoracic pressure, which results in increased systemic venous return and, if there is an unelastic pericardium encasing the heart, results in a rapid increase of the right heart pressures. Inspiration also results in decreased pulmonary vein return and, thus, a small drop in the left heart pressure. When there is constrictive physiology, these pressure differences result in an abrupt shift of the intraventricular septum leftwards. The septal shift is reversed during expiration, with restoration of the shape of the left ventricle. These pathophysiologic changes are best seen at the short-axis orientation during real-time imaging at deep inspiration and expiration. Additional information may be obtained with myocardial tagging, which can demonstrate adhesion of the thickened pericardium to the myocardium in patients with constrictive pericarditis [39].

27. A middle-aged woman is referred for a CMR study for evaluation of syncopal spells. The images in Fig. 4.33 are diastolic (left) and systolic (right) images from a cine functional study in the 4-chamber orientation. What is the likely diagnosis?

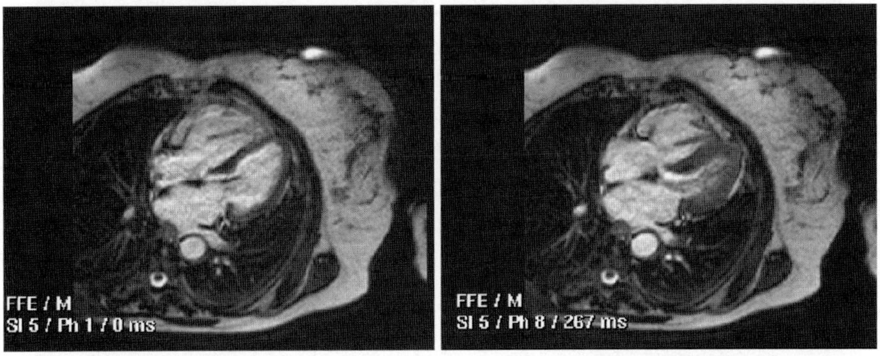

A. Hypertrophic cardiomyopathy
B. Infiltrative cardiomyopathy
C. Dilated cardiomyopathy
D. Arrhythmogenic right ventricular dysplasia
E. Atrial septal defect

Correct answer is D.

The images in Fig. 4.34 demonstrate dilation of the right ventricle (*RV*), with focal dyskinesis of the right ventricular free wall (*arrow*). The thickness of the left ventricular wall is normal without evidence of asymmetric hypertrophy, and the left ventricular systolic function is normal. The right atrium (*ra*) is normal in size, arguing against an atrial septal defect. Even if an atrial septal defect was present, it would not suffice to explain the right ventricular global and focal systolic dysfunction.

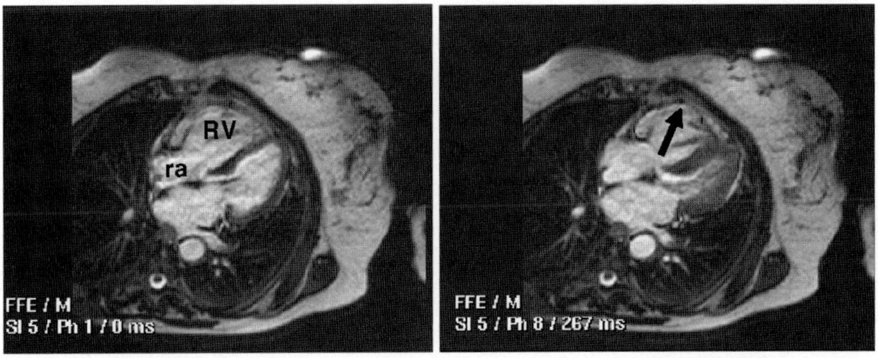

28. A 67-year-old man was noted to have an abnormal echocardiogram and was referred for a CMR study. The images in Fig. 4.35 are short-axis diastolic (A) and systolic (B) images from a cine functional study.

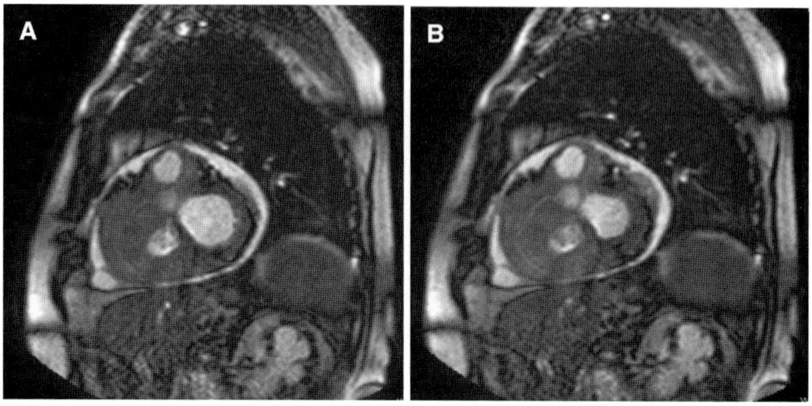

What is the likely diagnosis?

A. Normal study with image artifact
B. Severe right ventricular hypertrophy
C. Myxoma
D. Hypertrophic cardiomyopathy
E. Malignant cardiac tumor

Correct answer is E.

Figure 4.36 demonstrates a tissue with intermediate signal intensity that occupies most of the right atrioventricular groove (*A, black arrows*) and extends up to the root of the pulmonary artery (*A, white arrow*). This tissue appears to encase the right coronary artery (*B, arrowheads*). There is a circumferential pericardial effusion (bright rim around the heart). These findings are obviously not artifactual and cannot be attributed to hypertrophic cardiomyopathy. Right ventricular hypertrophy would not encase the right coronary artery, neither would it explain the pericardial effusion. Myxomas may occasionally be intramyocardial, but the invasion around the right coronary artery could not be explained. Thus, the CMR diagnosis is malignant cardiac tumor. Pathology revealed metastatic bladder adenocarcinoma. CMR cannot make a histological diagnosis; sarcoma, melanoma, or other malignant solid tumors could also provide the same picture and should be included in the differential diagnosis.

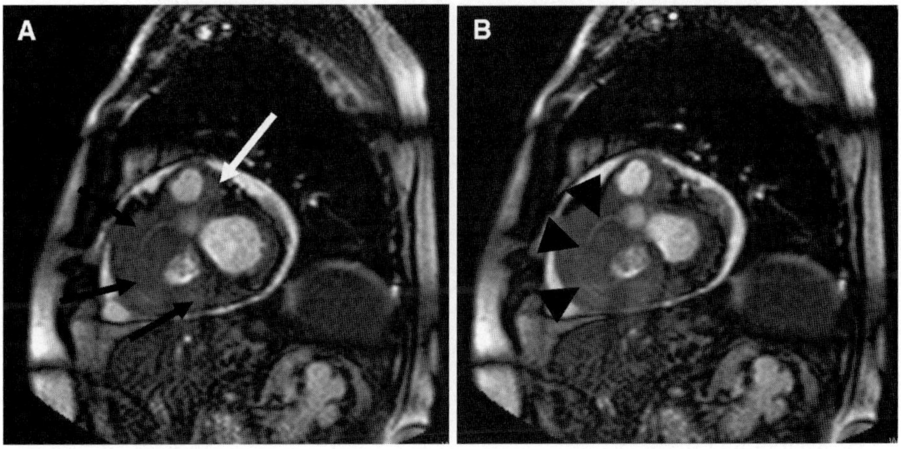

29. The images in Fig. 4.37 were obtained in a young competitive athlete who was noted to have an abnormal ECG. A, B, and C are images obtained in the transverse orientation. A is a T1-weighted image; B is a T1-weighted image after gadolinium enhancement; and C is a T2-weighted image. D and E are images obtained in the 4-chamber orientation. D is a diastolic image from a cine functional study and E is an image with heavy T1-weighting obtained late after contrast administration. What is the most likely diagnosis?

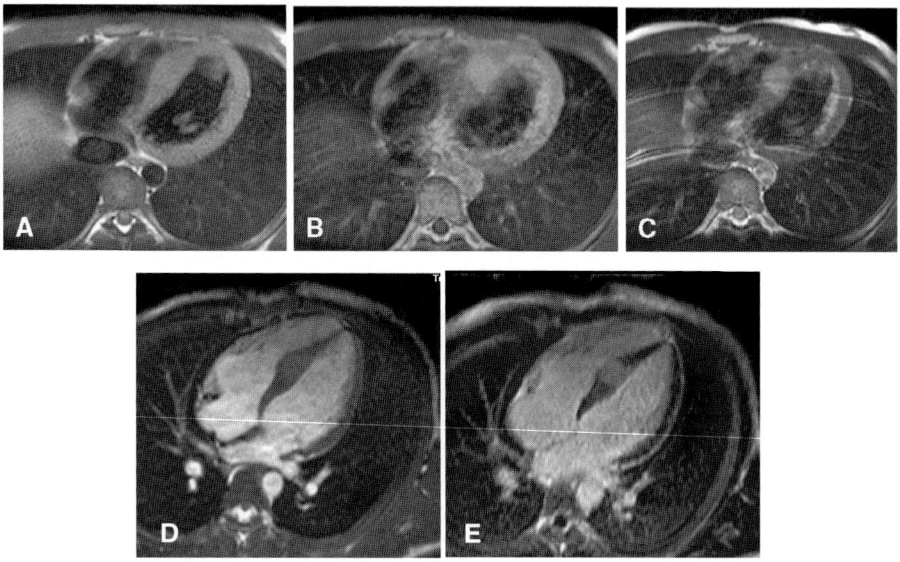

A. Hypertrophic cardiomyopathy
B. Lipomatous degeneration of the intraventricular septum
C. Intramyocardial hemangioma
D. Myxoma
E. Rhabdomyoma

Correct answer is C.

The images in Fig. 4.37 demonstrate replacement of the mid-portion of the intraventricular septum by a solid tissue that has signal intensity similar to the myocardium in T1-weighted images (*A*), but enhances more than the normal myocardium after contrast administration (*B*). This tissue has also higher signal (hyperintense) in the T2-weighted sequence (*C*) and retains contrast in the delayed images (*E*). All of these imaging characteristics are fairly typical for hemangiomas, and, despite the absence of histological confirmation in this case, the diagnosis can be made with a high degree of certainty based on the CMR study. The abnormal tissue does not have imaging characteristics of myocardium, therefore, excluding the possibility of hypertrophic cardiomyopathy and making the case of rhabdomyoma unlikely. Myxomas are almost always intracavitary structures. Finally, lipomatous degeneration of the intraventricular septum is highly unlikely, because the presence of adipose tissue would be readily apparent as high signal in the T1- and T2-weighted sequences (similar to subcutaneous fat).

30. Figure 4.38 shows diastolic (A) and systolic (B) images from a CMR study in a patient with grossly abnormal 12-lead ECG (tall R waves with deep inverted T waves in the precordial leads).

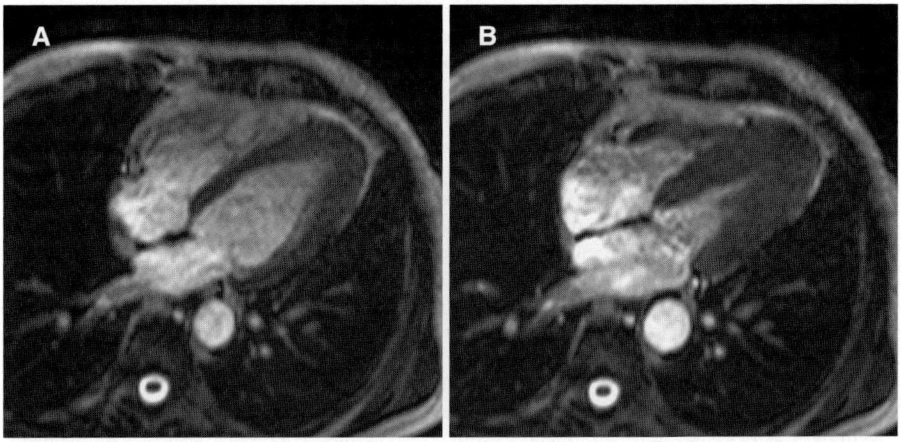

What is the most likely diagnosis?

A. Dilated cardiomyopathy
B. Hypertrophic obstructive cardiomyopathy
C. Apical hypertrophic cardiomyopathy (Yamaguchi)
D. Takotsubo cardiomyopathy
E. Noncompaction cardiomyopathy

Correct answer is C.

Apical hypertrophic cardiomyopathy is characterized by apical hypertrophy with normal wall thickness at the basal ventricular walls. Unlike the focal septal hypertrophy, apical hypertrophic cardiomyopathy does not cause outflow obstruction. CMR can define well the ventricular morphology and function in these patients [40] and compares favorably to echocardiography for assessment of the ventricular apex [41]. There is no evidence of dilated cardiomyopathy, apical ballooning (Takotsubo cardiomyopathy), or noncompaction of the left ventricle.

References

1. Frank H and Globits S. Magnetic resonance imaging evaluation of myocardial and pericardial disease. *J Magn Reson Imaging*, 1999;10(5):617–626.
2. Masui T, Finck S, and Higgins CB. Constrictive pericarditis and restrictive cardiomyopathy: evaluation with MR imaging. *Radiology*, 1992;182(2):369–373.
3. Sechtem U, Tscholakoff D, and Higgins CB. MRI of the abnormal pericardium. *AJR Am J Roentgenol*, 1986;147(2):245–252.
4. Sechtem U, Tscholakoff D, and Higgins CB. MRI of the normal pericardium. *AJR Am J Roentgenol*, 1986;147(2):239–244.
5. Codreanu A, Djaballah W, Angioi M, et al. Detection of myocarditis by contrast-enhanced MRI in patients presenting with acute coronary syndrome but no coronary stenosis. *J Magn Reson Imaging*, 2007;25(5):957–964.
6. Deetjen AG, Conradi G, Mollmann S, Rad A, Hamm CW, and Dill T. Value of gadolinium-enhanced magnetic resonance imaging in patients with Tako-Tsubo-like left ventricular dysfunction. *J Cardiovasc Magn Reson*, 2006;8(2):367–372.
7. Friedrich MG, Strohm O, Schulz-Menger J, Marciniak H, Luft FC, and Dietz R. Contrast media-enhanced magnetic resonance imaging visualizes myocardial changes in the course of viral myocarditis. *Circulation*, 1998;97(18):1802–1809.
8. Haghi D, Fluechter S, Suselbeck T, Borggrefe M, and Papavassiliu T. Delayed hyperenhancement in a case of Takotsubo cardiomyopathy. *J Cardiovasc Magn Reson*, 2005;7(5):845–847.
9. Laissy JP, Messin B, Varenne O, et al. MRI of acute myocarditis: a comprehensive approach based on various imaging sequences. *Chest*, 2002;122(5):1638–1648.
10. Roditi GH, Hartnell GG, and Cohen MC. MRI changes in myocarditis—evaluation with spin echo, cine MR angiography and contrast enhanced spin echo imaging. *Clin Radiol*, 2000;55(10):752–758.
11. Yelgec NS, Dymarkowski S, Ganame J, and Bogaert J. Value of MRI in patients with a clinical suspicion of acute myocarditis. *Eur Radiol*, 2007.
12. Luna A, Ribes R, Caro P, Vida J, and Erasmus JJ. Evaluation of cardiac tumors with magnetic resonance imaging. *Eur Radiol*, 2005;15(7):1446–1455.
13. Mozaffarian D and Caldwell JH. Right ventricular involvement in hypertrophic cardiomyopathy: a case report and literature review. *Clin Cardiol*, 2001;24(1):2–8.
14. Wang ZJ, Reddy GP, Gotway MB, Yeh BM, Hetts SW, and Higgins CB. CT and MR imaging of pericardial disease. *Radiographics*, 2003;23 Spec No:S167–180.
15. Maksimovic R, Dill T, Seferovic PM, et al. Magnetic resonance imaging in pericardial diseases. Indications and diagnostic value. *Herz*, 2006;31(7):708–714.
16. Francone M, Dymarkowski S, Kalantzi M, and Bogaert J. Real-time cine MRI of ventricular septal motion: a novel approach to assess ventricular coupling. *J Magn Reson Imaging*, 2005;21(3):305–309.
17. Giorgi B, Mollet NR, Dymarkowski S, Rademakers FE, and Bogaert J. Clinically suspected constrictive pericarditis: MR imaging assessment of ventricular septal motion and configuration in patients and healthy subjects. *Radiology*, 2003;228(2):417–424.
18. Fieno DS, Saouaf R, Thomson LE, Abidov A, Friedman JD, and Berman DS. Cardiovascular magnetic resonance of primary tumors of the heart: A review. *J Cardiovasc Magn Reson*, 2006;8(6):839–853.
19. Kaminaga T, Takeshita T, and Kimura I. Role of magnetic resonance imaging for evaluation of tumors in the cardiac region. *Eur Radiol*, 2003;13 Suppl 4:L1–10.
20. Sparrow PJ, Kurian JB, Jones TR, and Sivananthan MU. MR imaging of cardiac tumors. *Radiographics*, 2005;25(5):1255–1276.
21. Fertin M, Mouquet F, Lallemant R, et al. Diagnosis, imaging, and treatment of an unusual cardiac hydatid cyst. *Cardiovasc Pathol*, 2006;15(6):356–358.
22. Kotoulas GK, Magoufis GL, Gouliamos AD, et al. Evaluation of hydatid disease of the heart with magnetic resonance imaging. *Cardiovasc Intervent Radiol*, 1996;19(3):187–189.

23. Kiaffas MG, Powell AJ, and Geva T. Magnetic resonance imaging evaluation of cardiac tumor characteristics in infants and children. *Am J Cardiol*, 2002;89(10):1229–1233.
24. Rickers C, Wilke NM, Jerosch-Herold M, et al. Utility of cardiac magnetic resonance imaging in the diagnosis of hypertrophic cardiomyopathy. *Circulation*, 2005;112(6):855–861.
25. Petersen SE, Selvanayagam JB, Wiesmann F, et al. Left ventricular non-compaction: insights from cardiovascular magnetic resonance imaging. *J Am Coll Cardiol*, 2005;46(1):101–105.
26. Pennell DJ. T2* magnetic resonance and myocardial iron in thalassemia. *Ann N Y Acad Sci*, 2005;1054:373–378.
27. He T, Gatehouse PD, Anderson LJ, et al. Development of a novel optimized breathhold technique for myocardial T2 measurement in thalassemia. *J Magn Reson Imaging*, 2006;24(3):580–585.
28. Westwood M, Anderson LJ, Firmin DN, et al. A single breath-hold multiecho T2* cardiovascular magnetic resonance technique for diagnosis of myocardial iron overload. *J Magn Reson Imaging*, 2003;18(1):33–39.
29. Gotte MJ, Germans T, Russel IK, et al. Myocardial strain and torsion quantified by cardiovascular magnetic resonance tissue tagging: studies in normal and impaired left ventricular function. *J Am Coll Cardiol*, 2006;48(10):2002–2011.
30. Sueyoshi E, Sakamoto I, Okimoto T, Hayashi K, Tanaka K, and Toda G. Cardiac amyloidosis: typical imaging findings and diffuse myocardial damage demonstrated by delayed contrast-enhanced MRI. *Cardiovasc Intervent Radiol*, 2006;29(4):710–712.
31. Kwong RY and Falk RH. Cardiovascular magnetic resonance in cardiac amyloidosis. *Circulation*, 2005;111(2):122–124.
32. Maceira AM, Joshi J, Prasad SK, et al. Cardiovascular magnetic resonance in cardiac amyloidosis. *Circulation*, 2005;111(2):186–193.
33. Lembcke A, Meyer R, Kivelitz D, et al. Images in cardiovascular medicine. Papillary fibroelastoma of the aortic valve: appearance in 64-slice spiral computed tomography, magnetic resonance imaging, and echocardiography. *Circulation*, 2007;115(1):e3–6.
34. Isbell DC and Kramer CM. Magnetic resonance for the assessment of myocardial viability. *Curr Opin Cardiol*, 2006;21(5):469–472.
35. Kim DH, Choi SI, Chang HJ, Choi DJ, Lim C, and Park JH. Delayed hyperenhancement by contrast-enhanced magnetic resonance imaging: Clinical application for various cardiac diseases. *J Comput Assist Tomogr*, 2006;30(2):226–232.
36. Vogel-Claussen J, Rochitte CE, Wu KC, et al. Delayed enhancement MR imaging: utility in myocardial assessment. *Radiographics*, 2006;26(3):795–810.
37. Tandri H, Calkins H, Nasir K, et al. Magnetic resonance imaging findings in patients meeting task force criteria for arrhythmogenic right ventricular dysplasia. *J Cardiovasc Electrophysiol*, 2003;14(5):476–482.
38. van der Wall EE, Kayser HW, Bootsma MM, de Roos A, and Schalij MJ. Arrhythmogenic right ventricular dysplasia: MRI findings. *Herz*, 2000,25(4):356–364.
39. Kojima S, Yamada N, and Goto Y. Diagnosis of constrictive pericarditis by tagged cine magnetic resonance imaging. *N Engl J Med*, 1999;341(5):373–374.
40. Sperling RT, Parker JA, Manning WJ, and Danias PG. Apical hypertrophic cardiomyopathy: clinical, electrocardiographic, scintigraphic, echocardiographic, and magnetic resonance imaging findings of a case. *J Cardiovasc Magn Reson*, 2002;4(2):291–295.
41. Di Cesare E. MRI of the cardiomyopathies. *Eur J Radiol*, 2001;38(3):179–184.

5

Ischemic Heart Disease

Peter G. Danias, *Cardiovascular MRI: 150 Multiple-Choice Questions and Answers*

1. For CMR coronary angiography, data are typically obtained over several cardiac cycles. To freeze cardiac motion, it is desirable to obtain image data during a very short time period within each cycle.

What would the optimal time for data collection be?

A. 75 ms after the QRS
B. 150 ms after the QRS
C. Early diastole
D. Mid diastole
E. Late diastole

Correct answer is D.

Coronary motion is typically minimal during diastasis that occurs after rapid ventricular filling and before atrial filling, i.e., in mid diastole. End systole (typically occurring at 250–300 ms after the QRS) is another phase of relatively little cardiac motion [1, 2]. In certain individuals, and particularly those with fast heart rates and children, end systole may be more appropriate for coronary MR angiography, because, with tachycardia, the diastolic period, and particularly diastasis, significantly shortens. During the early phases of ventricular contraction (100–200 ms), there is fast displacement of the base of the heart toward the apex, whereas significant motion also occurs in the opposite direction during rapid ventricular filling (early diastole) and atrial filling (late diastole). Some protocols for coronary MR angiography recommend manual inspection of a cine loop (4-chamber or horizontal orientation) to identify the time of minimal coronary artery motion for and individualized selection of the optimal timing for data collection.

2. In a patient with ischemic cardiomyopathy, which of the following findings in a CMR study would *not* be expected?

A. Dilation of the left ventricle
B. Regional thinning of the left ventricular wall
C. Subendocardial delayed enhancement after contrast (gadolinium) administration, with sparing of the epicardium
D. Epicardial delayed enhancement after contrast (gadolinium) administration, with sparing of the subendocardium
E. Transmural enhancement after contrast (gadolinium) administration

Correct answer is D.

Ischemic cardiomyopathy is typically caused by previous myocardial infarctions, which cause left ventricular wall thinning and dilation of the left ventricle. Infarctions may be either subendocardial (non-ST elevation or non-Q) or transmural (ST elevation or Q-wave). The former can be visualized as subendocardial regions with delayed enhancement, whereas the latter present as transmural enhancement late after contrast administration. Epicardial enhancement with endocardial sparing is more typical of myocarditis and infiltrative cardiomyopathy and is not seen with ischemic heart disease [3–5].

3. Which of the following ions is increased in infarcted and scarred myocardium, allowing for ion-specific CMR evaluation?

A. Sodium
B. Potassium
C. Phosphorous
D. Hydrogen
E. Iron

Correct answer is A.

Potassium and phosphorous are at high concentrations inside the normal myocytes, the former because of the Na–K membrane pump and the latter because of active oxidative metabolism (ADP, ATP, etc). Hydrogen and iron are not measurably different in normal and infarcted territories. Sodium accumulates in the infarcted territories, and this is the basis for Na-23 imaging to identify scar tissue in the myocardium [6, 7]. High field (3 T) is preferable for Na-23 imaging, because of enhanced signal-to-noise ratio. However, even with conventional 1.5-T systems, sodium imaging of myocardial scar is feasible and has been reported.

4. A 49-year-old man has suffered a myocardial infarction, for which he was treated with intravenous thrombolysis 3 hours after the onset of symptoms. Six months later, he has left ventricular dysfunction with akinesis of the distal half of the anterior wall, intraventricular septum, and apex. CMR is performed to assess myocardial viability. Delayed imaging after gadolinium administration demonstrates hyperenhancement of 20% of the total wall thickness, in the subendocardial region of most of the distal distribution of the left anterior descending coronary artery. X-ray contrast angiography demonstrates 100% occlusion of the left anterior descending coronary artery in its mid portion, with left-to-left collaterals filling the distal segment. What is the likelihood of improvement of systolic function in the distal anterior wall, intraventricular septum, and apex if coronary revascularization were to be performed?

A. 5%
B. 10%
C. 20%
D. 35%
E. 50%

Correct answer is E.

Based on multiple studies, there is an almost linear relationship between likelihood of improvement of systolic function after revascularization and percent thickness of the scar (i.e., transmural extent of myocardial necrosis) after a myocardial infarction. Clinically, when the scar thickness is less than 50% (or 25% according to some) of the total wall thickness, there is a good chance (>50%) for improvement of regional systolic function with revascularization. This is true even for akinetic or dyskinetic regions [8].

5. Which of the following gadolinium doses is most appropriate for assessment of myocardial viability?

A. 0.01 mmol/kg
B. 0.2 mmol/kg
C. 0.5 mmol/kg
D. 1 mmol/kg
E. Standard dose of 100 mmol (not weight-based)

Correct answer is B.

The dose of gadolinium for assessment of myocardial viability is weight-adjusted. Most cardiac MRI centers administer "double dose," i.e., 0.2 mmol/kg, although a dose of 0.1 mmol/kg has also been described in the literature in protocols of assessment of myocardial viability.

6. Figure 5.1 is a delayed-enhanced image in the 4-chamber orientation from a patient with heart failure.

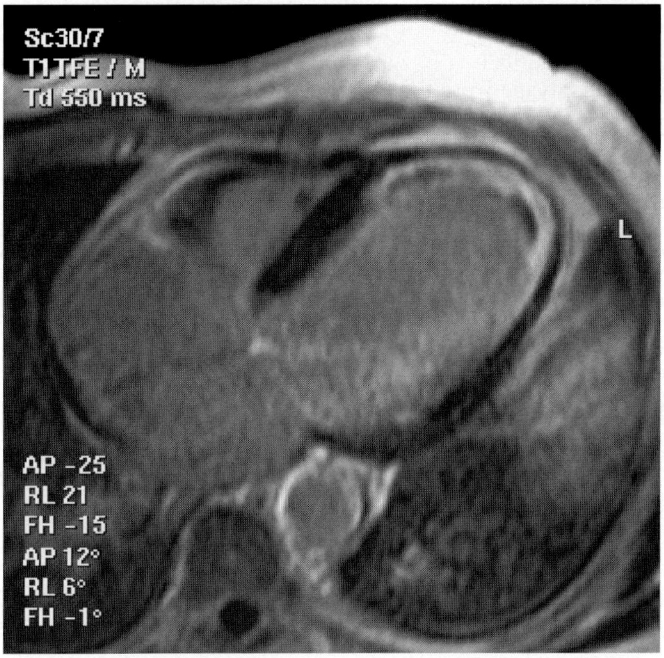

What is the likely diagnosis?

A. Nonischemic dilated cardiomyopathy
B. Hypertrophic cardiomyopathy
C. Restrictive cardiomyopathy
D. Constrictive pericarditis
E. Ischemic cardiomyopathy

Correct answer is E.

The left ventricle is dilated, arguing against hypertrophic or restrictive cardiomyopathy, or constrictive pericarditis. The apex and apical septal and lateral walls demonstrate almost transmural hyperenhancement that is consistent with scar in the distribution of the left anterior descending coronary artery.

7. In the patient described in Question 6, the dark rim at the endocardial surface of the apex is likely:

A. Mural thrombus
B. Incomplete myocardial signal suppression from incorrectly selected inversion time
C. Susceptibility artifact
D. Myocardial salvage from timely reperfusion therapy
E. Suggestive of noncompaction cardiomyopathy

Correct answer is A.

Chronic intracavitary thrombi do not take up contrast, because they are avascular structures. The typical appearance of a mural thrombus is a low-signal focal area attached to a scarred region (hyperintense in the delayed-enhanced images) [9]. Differential diagnosis should also include microvascular obstruction [10]; the separation may be difficult to make in cases in which there is only a thin dark rim lining the endocardium. With successful reperfusion therapy, myocardial salvage is first evident in the epicardial rather than the subendocardial regions. There is no evidence of incomplete myocardial signal suppression (normal myocardium appears black), of any susceptibility artifacts, or of noncompacted left ventricular myocardium.

8. Figure 5.2 is a single image form a delayed-enhanced study in the 2-chamber orientation at the midventricular level in an elderly patient scheduled to undergo cardiac surgery.

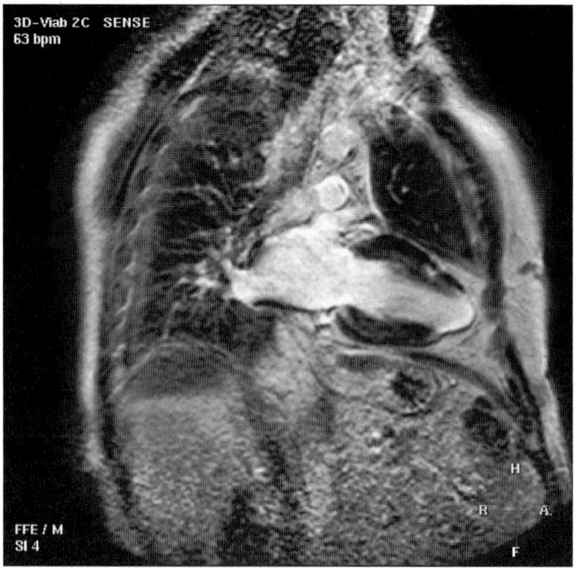

Which of the following statements is correct?

A. There is evidence of a myocardial infarction in the left anterior descending coronary artery distribution
B. There is evidence of a myocardial infarction in the left circumflex coronary artery distribution
C. There is evidence of a myocardial infarction in the right coronary artery distribution
D. There is evidence of a nontransmural myocardial infarction
E. There is no evidence of a myocardial infarction

Correct answer is A.

The image demonstrates apical wall thinning with transmural enhancement, consistent with myocardial scar. The location is fairly typical of a mid left anterior descending infarction and involves the distal anterior wall, apex, and inferoapical regions. Based on the transmural involvement of the hyperenhanced region and on the thickness of the apical wall, one would not expect functional recovery in the infarcted territory if revascularization were to be performed.

9. The images in Fig. 5.3 were obtained from a patient with coronary artery disease (CAD), heart failure, and pulmonary embolism. The image on the *left* is a diastolic frame from a 4-chamber study, and the image on the *right* is a delayed contrast-enhanced image at the same orientation.

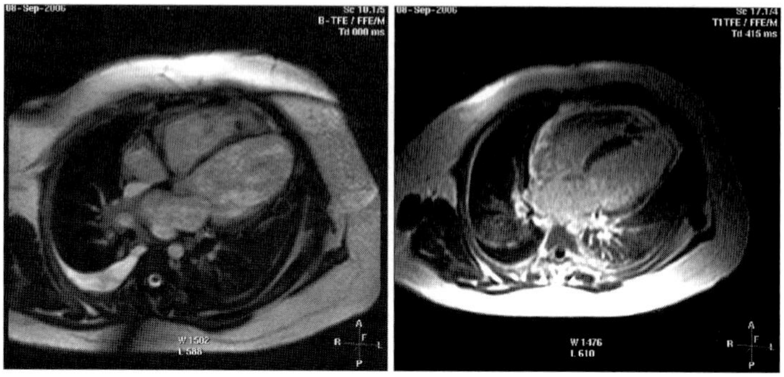

Which of the following pathologic findings is *not* present?

A. Left ventricular dilation
B. Apical infarct
C. Right pleural effusion
D. Right ventricular clot
E. Left ventricular apical clot

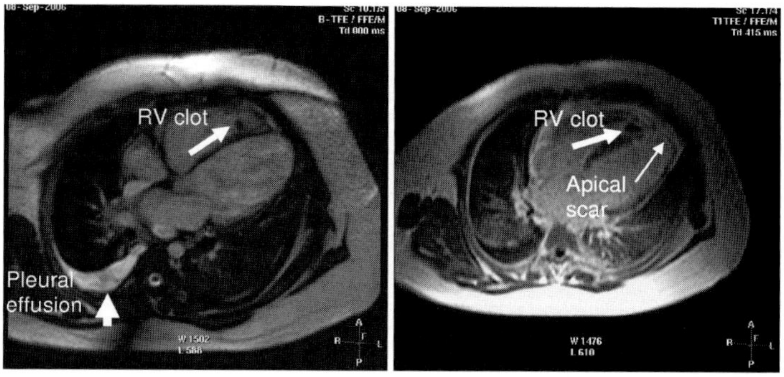

Correct answer is E.

The findings are noted in the images in Fig. 5.4. In both images, there is a round, well-circumscribed structure inside the right ventricular cavity (marked *RV clot*), which can be distinguished from the normal right ventricular trabeculations from the complete absence of signal (appears much darker than the ventricular wall) in the delayed contrast-enhanced images. The differential diagnosis of this structure would also include a vegetation, which is also an avascular structure and, thus, does not take up any contrast. The apical scar is transmural, because there is no viable myocardium surrounding the bright apical rim. There is no mural thrombus identified in the left ventricle.

10. In a patient with CAD undergoing CMR for evaluation of myocardial viability, delayed images are obtained after contrast is administered intravenously. This study demonstrates a dark endocardial rim adjacent to a bright transmural infarct zone. Which of the following would *not* be in the differential diagnosis of this finding?

A. Mural clot
B. Microvascular obstruction
C. Calcium deposition at the endocardial surface of the infarct territory
D. A combination of the above
E. Preserved endocardial viability with only epicardial extension of the infarct

Correct answer is E.

It is not possible to have preserved (viable) subendocardium with infarcted epicardium. Ischemia and infarction occur first at the subendocardial layers, because the coronary arteries end in the endocardium. Any compromise of coronary blood flow would first affect the distal vascular bed, i.e., the subendocardial layer. Delayed absence of contrast uptake can occur from microvascular obstruction, or within a mural clot (avascular structure). In old infarctions, calcium may be deposited on the infarct territory, causing loss of signal because of susceptibility artifact at the site of calcification.

11. In a patient with left ventricular dilation and severe systolic dysfunction, which of the following findings would be the *least* likely to distinguish between ischemic and nonischemic etiologies?

A. Regional systolic dysfunction
B. Presence of scar in the distribution of more than one coronary artery
C. Signal loss in the left main coronary artery at an MR coronary angiogram
D. Presence of an intracavitary left ventricular clot
E. Delayed rate of signal enhancement in the distribution of a coronary artery at first-pass gadolinium imaging

Correct answer is D.

In ischemic cardiomyopathy, the systolic dysfunction occurs at regions of the myocardium along the distribution of coronary arteries. Therefore, the presence of regional systolic dysfunction, the presence of scar, and the decreased perfusion at a coronary artery distribution suggest the presence of significant CAD, i.e., the ischemic etiology of cardiomyopathy. Similarly, MR coronary angiography is not considered as equivalent to the conventional X-ray coronary angiography, but, in the right context, the presence of signal loss in the proximal coronary arteries can suggest the ischemic etiology of cardiomyoapthy. The presence of intracavitary clots does not help distinguish ischemic from nonischemic cardiomyopathies, and clots may occur in both, when there is severe systolic dysfunction and slow blood flow.

12. A dobutamine stress CMR study is performed in a patient with decreased left ventricular systolic function to assess for the presence and extent of CAD as the etiology of the cardiomyopathy. Which of the following suggests the presence of significant coronary disease with considerable myocardial viability?

A. Augmentation of global systolic function at 5, 10, and 40 μg/kg/min
B. Decrease of systolic function at low-dose dobutamine (5–10 μg/kg/min) with augmentation of systolic function at higher dobutamine doses
C. Augmentation of global systolic function at low-dose dobutamine (5–10 μg/kg/min) with regional systolic dysfunction at higher dobutamine doses
D. Decrease of regional and global systolic function at low dose dobutamine (5–10 μg/kg/min)
E. None of the above. It would not be appropriate to perform CMR in such a patient

Correct answer is C.

Augmentation of systolic function at low-dose dobutamine followed by deterioration of regional (and global) systolic function is the classic "biphasic response," also described in dobutamine echocardiography [11–13]. At low doses of dobutamine administration, viable myocardium is recruited and augments its systolic performance. At higher doses of dobutamine, however, myocardial ischemia ensues because of the increased cardiac workload and regional function deteriorates. The augmentation of systolic function at both low and high dobutamine doses would suggest the nonischemic etiology of cardiomyoapthy. On the other hand, decrease of systolic function at even low-dose dobutamine would argue against the presence of significant myocardial viability. Dobutamine CMR is an accepted modality to test for the presence of CAD and assessment of viability.

13. Which of the following is the most appropriate statement regarding the clinical value of CMR coronary angiography for evaluation of aortocoronary bypass grafts?

A. CMR has no value for evaluation of bypass grafts
B. CMR has high sensitivity for the assessment of bypass patency, but has little clinical value for the evaluation of stenoses
C. CMR can accurately assess bypass graft patency and also the presence of significant stenoses
D. CMR can accurately assess bypass graft patency in the arterial but not the saphenous venous grafts
E. CMR is a substitute for conventional X-ray coronary angiography for the evaluation of bypass grafts

Correct answer is B.

In multiple studies, CMR has been shown to have high sensitivity for assessment of bypass graft patency, using black blood, white blood, and contrast-enhanced sequences [14]. For assessment of graft stenoses, however, CMR has similar performance to that for native coronary arteries, with intermediate–high sensitivity and intermediate specificity, both for the saphenous venous and internal mammary arterial grafts [15]. CMR is, therefore, not a substitute for conventional X-ray angiography for evaluation of bypass grafts, but does have some value when the question is only regarding graft patency.

14. With dobutamine stress CMR, which of the following statements is correct?

A. The inotropic reserve at low-dose dobutamine is a measure of myocardial ischemia
B. Baseline atrial fibrillation makes the study unreliable
C. Previous use of β-blockers does not interfere with the diagnostic accuracy for assessment of ischemia
D. In patients with left bundle branch block, wall thickening is unreliable as a criterion for assessment of myocardial inotropic reserve
E. Diagnostic accuracy is superior to that of dobutamine echocardiography

Correct answer is E.

Dobutamine CMR has been shown to have superior diagnostic accuracy compared with dobutamine echocardiography, because of improved image quality and endocardial border definition of all myocardial regions. The inotropic reserve at low-dose dobutamine is a measure of myocardial viability but not of ischemia. Baseline atrial fibrillation makes the study difficult but not unreliable, because it affects mainly the diastolic and not the systolic period. As with dobutamine echocardiography [16] and dobutamine nuclear scintigraphy [17], the use of β-blockers likely decreases the sensitivity of dobutamine CMR for detection of ischemia. In patients with left bundle branch block, the wall motion may be unreliable for assessment of regional function because of the abnormal activation of the left ventricle. However, despite the conduction abnormality, the presence of wall thickening is thought to be a good measure of regional systolic function and inotropic augmentation with dobutamine.

15. Which of the following statements is correct regarding the usefulness of CMR coronary angiography?

A. It is indicated to assess for significant CAD
B. It is indicated for screening of subclinical atherosclerosis
C. It has high specificity but low–moderate sensitivity for detection of proximal significant CAD in selected individuals
D. It has high sensitivity but low–moderate specificity for detection of proximal and mid-significant CAD in selected individuals
E. It is not useful for assessment of coronary anomalies

Correct answer is D.

In multiple studies, CMR coronary angiography has been shown to have high sensitivity but low–moderate specificity for assessment of significant proximal coronary atherosclerosis [18, 19]. At the present time, CMR coronary angiography is not indicated for assessment of CAD or for the preclinical screening of coronary atherosclerosis. CMR can accurately assess the origin and proximal course of the coronary arteries and, thus, has clinical value for evaluation of coronary anomalies [20].

16. Which of the following statements regarding perfusion stress CMR is correct?

A. Imaging is performed at the time of injection of gadolinium (first pass), to assess for contrast delivery to the myocardium
B. Imaging is performed a few minutes after gadolinium administration, to assess for the early washout of the contrast
C. Imaging is performed a few minutes after gadolinium administration, to assess for the peak myocardial signal enhancement
D. Imaging is performed several minutes after gadolinium administration to assess for cellular uptake of gadolinium
E. Imaging is performed several minutes after gadolinium administration to assess for the late washout of the contrast

Correct answer is A.

Perfusion CMR depends on the first-pass imaging of gadolinium at the myocardium. The myocardial signal intensity change over time (in relation to the signal intensity in the left ventricular cavity) provides information regarding the delivery of the contrast agent via the coronary arteries. In multiple studies, stress perfusion CMR has been shown to be highly accurate for detection of CAD [21–29]. Gadolinium-based contrast media are extracellular agents that quickly diffuse into the interstitial space and are not taken up by the myocardial cells. In normal myocardium, gadolinium contrast is quickly washed out of the interstitial space in a matter of minutes. Delayed imaging after contrast administration is performed for assessment of myocardial viability and not for evaluation of perfusion.

17. Which of the following indices best describes myocardial perfusion using first-pass gadolinium imaging?

A. Peak left ventricular signal enhancement
B. Peak myocardial signal enhancement
C. Contrast arrival time to the myocardium
D. Time to peak signal enhancement
E. Slope of myocardial signal enhancement

Correct answer is E.

Peak myocardial signal enhancement, contrast arrival time, time to peak enhancement, and slope of myocardial signal enhancement at first pass have all been described as parameters related to myocardial perfusion. Of all of these indices, the slope of myocardial signal enhancement is considered the most representative of myocardial perfusion [30]. The pattern of signal increase in the left ventricle provides information regarding the contrast bolus injection and is also considered during data analysis, but does not provide information regarding myocardial perfusion.

18. A patient with severe two-vessel CAD undergoes vasodilation perfusion CMR. Which of the following would be the expected finding?

A. Subendocardial hypoperfusion will result in apparent cavity dilation
B. Increased pulmonary uptake is a measure of severity of CAD
C. There will be a relative increase of the slope of signal enhancement after vasodilation in the territory that is supplied by the normal coronary artery, whereas, for the other territories, there will be decrease or no change of the slope of signal enhancement after vasodilation
D. All coronary territories will demonstrate a decrease of the slope of signal enhancement after vasodilation. The territory supplied by the normal coronary artery will have a slightly lower slope of myocardial signal enhancement compared with the other vascular territories
E. ECG changes during vasodilation are very sensitive in detection of severe CAD

Correct answer is C.

With perfusion CMR, the slope of signal enhancement is examined and the rest versus vasodilation patterns are compared. With normal epicardial coronary arteries, there is an increase of blood flow after vasodilation, resulting in an increase of the rate (slope) of myocardial signal enhancement. For severely diseased coronary arteries, one would expect a decrease or little change in the slope of signal enhancement at vasodilation at the corresponding territories [27]. The apparent cavity dilation and increased lung uptake are indirect findings suggestive of severe/multi-vessel CAD for radioisotopic myocardial perfusion imaging. ECG changes during vasodilation are an insensitive but highly specific marker of severe CAD, but usually cannot be assessed inside the CMR environment because of distortion of the surface ECG from the magnetohydrodynamic effect.

19. Figure 5.5 is a single short-axis image obtained with an inversion-recovery sequence 15 minutes after 0.2 mmol/kg Gd-DTPA administration in a patient with severe dyspnea on exertion. Which of the following statements best describes the findings of this image?

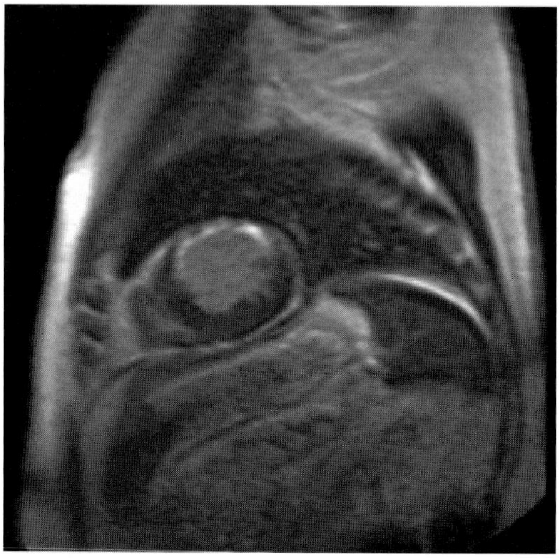

A. There is anterior and anterolateral wall scarring without significant myocardial viability in the infarct territory
B. There is anterior and anterolateral wall scarring with mostly viable myocardium in the infarct territory
C. There is extensive inferior, inferoseptal, and inferolateral wall scarring without myocardial viability in the infarct territory
D. There is extensive inferior, inferoseptal, and inferolateral wall scarring with mostly viable myocardium in the infarct territory
E. The patient has nonischemic cardiomyopathy

Correct answer is A.

Late gadolinium enhancement occurs in the infarct territory because of an increase of the extracellular space (volume of distribution) and a decrease of the washout of the contrast agent resulting from decreased blood flow. In the image presented, there is anterior and anterolateral wall scarring (bright region). Myocardial viability is suggested when the scar is nontransmural, i.e., less than 50% (or 25%) of the wall thickness [8]. In this case, the scar is near transmural, suggesting the absence of myocardial viability in the infarct territory.

20. Which of the following statements is correct regarding contrast-enhanced CMR coronary angiography?

A. Extracellular contrast agents (gadolinium chelates) have been approved since 2000 by the US Food and Drug Administration (FDA) for coronary artery CMR angiography because of superior vessel delineation, particularly with free-breathing techniques
B. Intravascular contrast agents have been approved since 2000 by the USFDA for coronary artery CMR angiography because of superior vessel delineation, particularly with breath-holding techniques
C. Up until 2004, no contrast media were USFDA approved for coronary CMR angiography
D. Paramagnetic contrast media significantly increase the blood T1, allowing for superior delineation of the coronary vessels
E. Contrast-enhanced CMR coronary angiography with intravascular contrast media has no potential for imaging of the atherosclerotic plaque, because the contrast remains only in the intravascular compartment

Correct answer is C.

Although commonly practiced in the clinical setting, contrast-enhanced MR angiography has not been approved by the USFDA at the time of writing of this textbook. In October 2005, the European Medicines Agency granted marketing approval of the intravascular gadolinium-based agent, Gadofosveset trisodium or MS-325 (Vasovist®, Epix Pharmaceuticals, Inc., Cambridge, MA) for all 25 member states of the European Union [31]. Intravascular agents have the greatest value for use with free-breathing approaches, in which the merits of sequences with longer imaging times can be exploited. Conversely, extracellular contrast agents have the greatest value for use with breath-holding approaches, in which imaging needs to be completed quickly, before the extravasation of the contrast to the interstitium. Paramagnetic contrast media decrease the T1 of the blood pool, allowing for better contrast-to-noise ratios and, thus, better delineation of the blood vessels. Intravascular contrast media have been reported to be promising for atherosclerotic plaque imaging. In the atherosclerotic plaque, signal enhancement after contrast administration is thought to be due to increased neovascularization.

21. An asymptomatic patient with suspected CAD because of a mild inferior defect at stress nuclear imaging, undergoes perfusion stress CMR at stress and rest. On the stress (vasodilation) image, a single territory at the inferior and inferoseptal walls demonstrates decreased endocardial signal with normal signal enhancement pattern at rest. Which of the following would be the most appropriate conclusion based on the findings of this study?

A. The patient has likely single-vessel disease—the right coronary artery most likely has a significant stenosis
B. The patient likely has no significant CAD. The apparent inferior defect in both nuclear and CMR images is most likely caused by diaphragmatic attenuation
C. The patient has likely nonischemic cardiomyopathy. Inferior defects are common in patients with cardiomyopathies
D. The patient should immediately undergo diagnostic coronary catheterization and angioplasty
E. An assessment of myocardial viability should be the next test, before invasive confirmation of CAD is entertained

Correct answer is A.

One of the advantages of perfusion CMR is that evaluation of each region is performed independently and not relative to other myocardial walls/segments. A subendocardial stress perfusion abnormality suggests CAD in the corresponding vessel (in this case, the right coronary artery). In patients with multivessel coronary disease, more than one myocardial wall/segment would be expected to have decreased signal of the subendocardial layer at stress. Diaphragmatic (inferior) attenuation is frequently an issue with nuclear myocardial perfusion imaging, particularly in patients with cardiomyopathy [32], but not with perfusion CMR. CMR has been reported to distinguish true from false-positive nuclear scan results in patients with inferior defects [33]. The decision to proceed with diagnostic cardiac catheterization and revascularization is a clinical one and would likely not be appropriate for this asymptomatic patient with single-vessel coronary disease. Evaluation for myocardial viability would not be indicated in this patient with a normal CMR myocardial perfusion pattern at rest.

22. The images in Fig. 5.6 are diastolic (*A*) and systolic (*B*) frames of a cine study of a middle-aged man with diabetes and shortness of breath. Which is the most likely diagnosis?

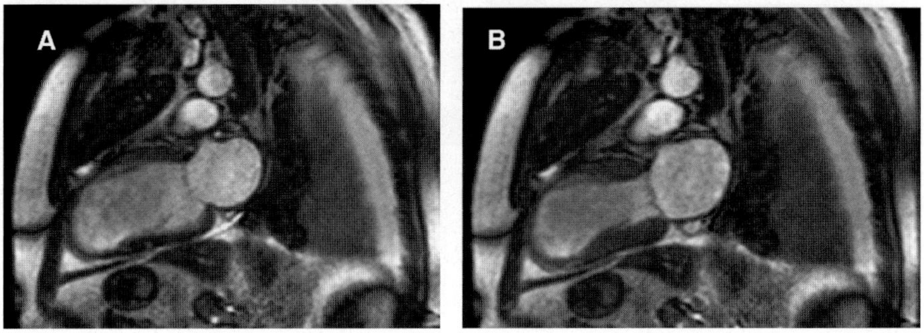

A. Ischemic cardiomyopathy with anterior and apical myocardial infarction
B. Nonischemic (diabetic) cardiomyopathy with predominantly apical involvement
C. Acute myocarditis with apical involvement
D. Takotsubo cardiomyopathy
E. Acute pulmonary embolism

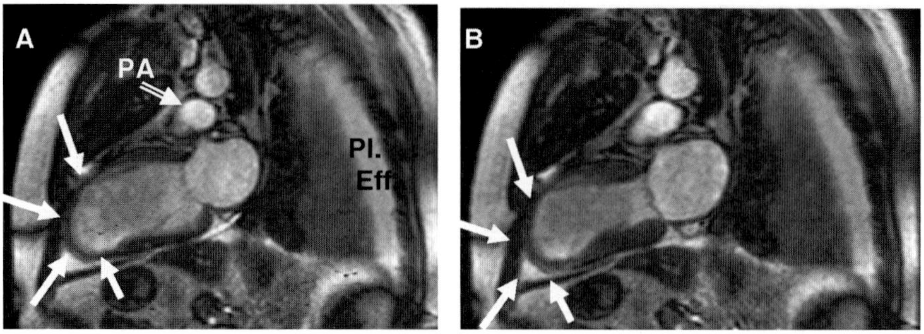

Correct answer is A.

In Fig. 5.7, in the diastolic frame (*A*), there is distal anterior, apical, and inferoapical wall thinning (*white solid arrows*). This is the typical distribution of the left anterior descending coronary artery. The systolic frame (*B*) demonstrates dyskinesis of the anteroapical region. Both of these findings are typical for ischemic cardiomyopathy after a large anteroapical myocardial infarction. Acute myocarditis with regional involvement is characterized by a focal wall motion abnormality with preserved wall thickness. Takotsubo cardiomyopathy is a rare form of acute cardiac involvement characterized by apical ballooning and wall thinning, usually occurring in women with minimal or no risk factors for CAD and precipitated by a severe emotional stressor event [34, 35]. Thus, although Takotsubo cardiomyoapthy should be considered in the differential diagnosis, with the clinical scenario provided here, ischemic cardiomyopathy would be the overwhelmingly more likely diagnosis. The diameter of the pulmonary artery (*PA*) appears normal, suggesting that pulmonary embolism is not the most likely diagnosis, particularly given the findings from the left ventricle. A large pleural effusion (*Pl.Eff.*) is also evident.

23. A gradient echo (bright blood) sequence is used to obtain a CMR coronary angiogram in a patient with known proximal right coronary artery occlusion and a previous inferior wall myocardial infarction. The presence of bright signal in the entire distal right coronary artery could occur in all of the following circumstances *except* for:

A. Right-to-right collaterals
B. Left-to-right collaterals
C. Recanalization of the infarct artery
D. Artifact caused by heavy vessel wall calcification
E. Bypass grafting of the posterior descending coronary artery

Correct answer is D.

The presence of bright signal suggestive of flow beyond a total coronary artery occlusion suggests that there is distal antegrade or retrograde blood flow. This can occur with collaterals, bypass graft surgery, or with recanalization of the infarct-related artery. Heavy calcification would cause susceptibility artifacts and signal loss rather than bright signal at the course of the coronary artery.

24. A patient with atrial fibrillation and wide RR variability is referred for a CMR study of the origin and proximal course of the coronary vessels for suspected coronary anomaly. Assuming that the imaging sequence has a temporal resolution of 70 ms, what would the optimal delay from the QRS onset be for obtaining a high-quality coronary scan?

A. 50 ms
B. 150 ms
C. 250 ms
D. 500 ms
E. As long as possible

Correct answer is C.

There are two points in the cardiac cycle with relatively little coronary artery motion. The first point is during mid-diastole, at diastasis, just after the rapid filling phase and before the atrial contraction. The second point is at peak systole [1, 2, 36]. With varying cycle length (i.e. RR interval), the systolic period remains relatively constant, while ventricular diastole is considerably affected and can vary widely. Therefore, mid-diastole occurs at a different time point after the onset of the QRS for each heartbeat. Accordingly, diastolic coronary artery imaging is unreliable and image artifacts invariably occur. This is the reason why, for these patients (as well as those with significant tachycardia, i.e., short-diastolic period), the preferred timing for coronary imaging is at end systole, which usually occurs approximately 250 ms after the onset of the QRS complex.

25. Dobutamine stress CMR compares favorably with dobutamine stress echocardiography for all the following reasons *except* for:

A. Ability to image obese patients and those with emphysema
B. Superior endocardial definition
C. Better patient monitoring
D. Highly reproducible imaging at the various levels of stress
E. Ability to combine with perfusion and scar imaging

Correct answer is C.

Dobutamine stress CMR has been reported to have higher sensitivity, specificity, and accuracy than dobutamine stress echocardiography, because of superior endocardial definition [37, 38]. Dobutamine stress CMR can image patients who are unsuitable for echocardiography because of poor acoustic windows (e.g., obese, patients with emphysema, etc.) with high degrees of accuracy [39]. With CMR, exactly the same orientations can be acquired at different levels of stress without the need for operator involvement, allowing for highly reproducible imaging. Perfusion and scar (viability) imaging can be combined with dobutamine stress CMR for better detection of CAD [40]. Patient monitoring is more difficult in the CMR environment, and claustrophobia is an additional limitation.

References

1. Al-Kwifi O, Stainsby J, Foltz WD, Sussman MS, Huang Y, and Wright GA. Characterizing coronary motion and its effect on MR coronary angiography—initial experience. *J Magn Reson Imaging*, 2006;24(4):842–850.
2. Wang Y, Watts R, Mitchell I, et al. Coronary MR angiography: selection of acquisition window of minimal cardiac motion with electrocardiography-triggered navigator cardiac motion prescanning—initial results. *Radiology*, 2001;218(2):580–585.
3. Jackson E, Bellenger N, Seddon M, Harden S, and Peebles C. Ischaemic and non-ischaemic cardiomyopathies—cardiac MRI appearances with delayed enhancement. *Clin Radiol*, 2007;62(5):395–403.
4. McCrohon JA, Moon JC, Prasad SK, et al. Differentiation of heart failure related to dilated cardiomyopathy and coronary artery disease using gadolinium-enhanced cardiovascular magnetic resonance. *Circulation*, 2003;108(1):54–59.
5. Wu E, Judd RM, Vargas JD, Klocke FJ, Bonow RO, and Kim RJ. Visualisation of presence, location, and transmural extent of healed Q-wave and non-Q-wave myocardial infarction. *Lancet*, 2001;357(9249):21–28.
6. Horn M. 23Na magnetic resonance imaging for the determination of myocardial viability: the status and the challenges. *Curr Vasc Pharmacol*, 2004;2(4):329–333.
7. Kim RJ, Judd RM, Chen EL, Fieno DS, Parrish TB, and Lima JA. Relationship of elevated 23Na magnetic resonance image intensity to infarct size after acute reperfused myocardial infarction. *Circulation*, 1999;100(2):185–192.
8. Kim RJ, Wu E, Rafael A, et al. The use of contrast-enhanced magnetic resonance imaging to identify reversible myocardial dysfunction. *N Engl J Med*, 2000;343(20):1445–1453.

9. Mollet NR, Dymarkowski S, Volders W, et al. Visualization of ventricular thrombi with contrast-enhanced magnetic resonance imaging in patients with ischemic heart disease. *Circulation*, 2002;106(23):2873–2876.
10. Hombach V, Grebe O, Merkle N, et al. Sequelae of acute myocardial infarction regarding cardiac structure and function and their prognostic significance as assessed by magnetic resonance imaging. *Eur Heart J*, 2005;26(6):549–557.
11. Hernandez-Pampaloni M, Peral V, Carreras JL, Sanchez-Harguindey L, and Vilacosta I. Biphasic response to dobutamine predicts improvement of left ventricular dysfunction after revascularization: correlation with positron emission and rest-redistribution 201Tl tomographies. *Int J Cardiovasc Imaging*, 2003;19(6):519–528.
12. Lancellotti P, Hoffer EP, and Pierard LA. Detection and clinical usefulness of a biphasic response during exercise echocardiography early after myocardial infarction. *J Am Coll Cardiol*, 2003;41(7):1142–1147.
13. Senior R and Lahiri A. Enhanced detection of myocardial ischemia by stress dobutamine echocardiography utilizing the "biphasic" response of wall thickening during low and high dose dobutamine infusion. *J Am Coll Cardiol*, 1995;26(1):26–32.
14. van Rossum AC, Galjee MA, Doesburg T, Hofman M, and Valk J. The role of magnetic resonance in the evaluation of functional results after CABG/PTCA. *Int J Card Imaging*, 1993;9 Suppl 1:59–69.
15. Langerak SE, Vliegen HW, de Roos A, et al. Detection of vein graft disease using high-resolution magnetic resonance angiography. *Circulation*, 2002;105(3):328–333.
16. Weissman NJ, Levangie MW, Guerrero JL, Weyman AE, and Picard MH. Effect of beta-blockade on dobutamine stress echocardiography. *Am Heart J*, 1996;131(4):698–703.
17. Shehata AR, Gillam LD, Mascitelli VA, et al. Impact of acute propranolol administration on dobutamine-induced myocardial ischemia as evaluated by myocardial perfusion imaging and echocardiography. *Am J Cardiol*, 1997;80(3):268–272.
18. Danias PG, Roussakis A, and Ioannidis JP. Diagnostic performance of coronary magnetic resonance angiography as compared against conventional X-ray angiography: a meta-analysis. *J Am Coll Cardiol*, 2004;44(9):1867–1876.
19. Kim WY, Danias PG, Stuber M, et al. Coronary magnetic resonance angiography for the detection of coronary stenoses. *N Engl J Med*, 2001;345(26):1863–1869.
20. Danias PG, Stuber M, McConnell MV, and Manning WJ. The diagnosis of congenital coronary anomalies with magnetic resonance imaging. *Coron Artery Dis*, 2001;12(8):621–626.
21. Crean A and Merchant N. MR perfusion and delayed enhancement imaging in the heart. *Clin Radiol*, 2006;61(3):225–236.
22. Croisille P, Revel D, and Saeed M. Contrast agents and cardiac MR imaging of myocardial ischemia: from bench to bedside. *Eur Radiol*, 2006;16(9):1951–1963.
23. Pennell DJ. Cardiovascular magnetic resonance and the role of adenosine pharmacologic stress. *Am J Cardiol*, 2004;94(2A):26D–31D; discussion 31D–32D.
24. Prasad SK, Lyne J, Chai P, and Gatehouse P. Role of CMR in assessment of myocardial perfusion. *Eur Radiol*, 2005;15 Suppl 2:B42–47.
25. Nagel E, al-Saadi N, and Fleck E. Cardiovascular magnetic resonance: myocardial perfusion. *Herz*, 2000;25(4):409–416.
26. Cury RC, Cattani CA, Gabure LA, et al. Diagnostic performance of stress perfusion and delayed-enhancement MR imaging in patients with coronary artery disease. *Radiology*, 2006;240(1):39–45.
27. Nagel E, Klein C, Paetsch I, et al. Magnetic resonance perfusion measurements for the noninvasive detection of coronary artery disease. *Circulation*, 2003;108(4):432–437.
28. Ishida N, Sakuma H, Motoyasu M, et al. Noninfarcted myocardium: correlation between dynamic first-pass contrast-enhanced myocardial MR imaging and quantitative coronary angiography. *Radiology*, 2003;229(1):209–216.
29. Schwitter J. Myocardial perfusion imaging by cardiac magnetic resonance. *J Nucl Cardiol*, 2006;13(6):841–854.

30. Al-Saadi N, Nagel E, Gross M, et al. Noninvasive detection of myocardial ischemia from perfusion reserve based on cardiovascular magnetic resonance. *Circulation*, 2000;101(12):1379–1383.
31. European Medicines Agency (EMEA). http://www.emea.europa.eu/humandocs/PDFs/EPAR/vasovist/060105en6.pdf, 2005.
32. Danias PG, Ahlberg AW, Clark BA, 3rd, et al. Combined assessment of myocardial perfusion and left ventricular function with exercise technetium-99m sestamibi gated single-photon emission computed tomography can differentiate between ischemic and nonischemic dilated cardiomyopathy. *Am J Cardiol*, 1998;82(10):1253–1258.
33. McCrohon JA, Lyne JC, Rahman SL, Lorenz CH, Underwood SR, and Pennell DJ. Adjunctive role of cardiovascular magnetic resonance in the assessment of patients with inferior attenuation on myocardial perfusion SPECT. *J Cardiovasc Magn Reson*, 2005;7(2):377–382.
34. Deetjen AG, Conradi G, Mollmann S, Rad A, Hamm CW, and Dill T. Value of gadolinium-enhanced magnetic resonance imaging in patients with Tako-Tsubo-like left ventricular dysfunction. *J Cardiovasc Magn Reson*, 2006;8(2):367–372.
35. Nef HM, Mollmann H, Kostin S, et al. Tako-Tsubo cardiomyopathy: intraindividual structural analysis in the acute phase and after functional recovery. *Eur Heart J*, 2007;28(20):2456–2464.
36. Shechter G, Resar JR, and McVeigh ER. Rest period duration of the coronary arteries: implications for magnetic resonance coronary angiography. *Med Phys*, 2005;32(1):255–262.
37. Nagel E, Lehmkuhl HB, Bocksch W, et al. Noninvasive diagnosis of ischemia-induced wall motion abnormalities with the use of high-dose dobutamine stress MRI: comparison with dobutamine stress echocardiography. *Circulation*, 1999;99(6):763–770.
38. Mandapaka S and Hundley WG. Dobutamine cardiovascular magnetic resonance: a review. *J Magn Reson Imaging*, 2006;24(3):499–512.
39. Hundley WG, Hamilton CA, Thomas MS, et al. Utility of fast cine magnetic resonance imaging and display for the detection of myocardial ischemia in patients not well suited for second harmonic stress echocardiography. *Circulation*, 1999;100(16):1697–1702.
40. Rerkpattanapipat P, Link KM, Hamilton CA, and Hundley WG. Clinical utility of assessments of left ventricular systolic function and coronary arterial blood flow during pharmacological stress with magnetic resonance imaging. *Top Magn Reson Imaging*, 2000;11(6):399–405.

6

Congenital Heart Disease

Peter G. Danias, *Cardiovascular MRI: 150 Multiple-Choice Questions and Answers*

1. The image in Fig. 6.1 is a planar reconstruction of a cardiovascular magnetic resonance imaging (CMR) coronary angiogram.

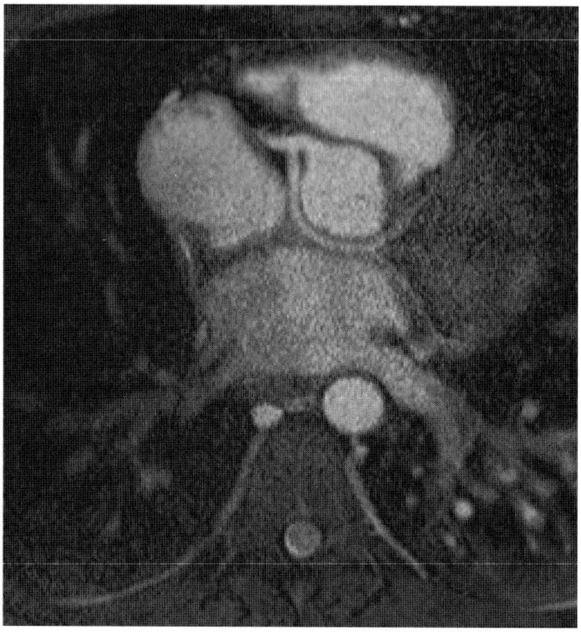

The diagnosis is:

A. Normal coronary anatomy
B. Anomalous takeoff of the right coronary artery
C. Anomalous takeoff of the left anterior descending coronary artery
D. Anomalous takeoff of the left circumflex coronary artery
E. Anomalous takeoff of the left coronary artery

Correct answer is E.

The coronary arteries are labeled in Figure 6.2. The right coronary artery (*RCA*) takes off from the right sinus of Valsalva with an anterior orientation, as usual. The left coronary artery (left main, *LM*) takes off from the right coronary artery and courses behind the aorta (benign form of coronary anomaly). The left anterior descending (*LAD*) and left circumflex (*LCx*) coronary arteries take off from the left main artery and course along the anterior intraventricular groove and left atrioventricular groove, as usual. The right ventricular outflow tract (*RVOT*), right atrium (*RA*), left atrium (*LA*), aortic root (*Ao*), and descending thoracic aorta (*DAo*) are also labeled. CMR is considered the best modality to evaluate the origin and proximal course of the coronary arteries [1].

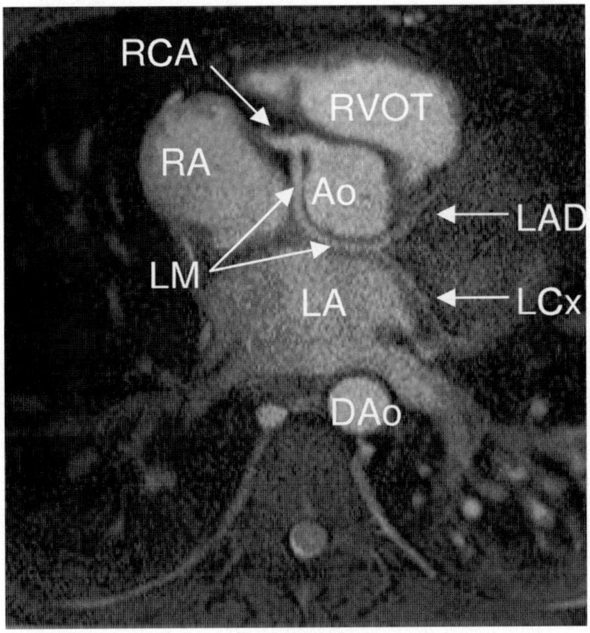

2. A 20-year-old acyanotic patient is referred for CMR because of a murmur and abnormal echocardiogram. The flows of the systemic and pulmonic circulation are measured using a phase-contrast sequence in planes perpendicular to the aorta and pulmonary trunk immediately distal to the semilunar valves. The Qp/Qs was measured at 0.6. The images that would establish the diagnosis are:

A. A phase-contrast scan obtained along the intra-atrial septum
B. A phase-contrast scan obtained along the intraventricular septum
C. Contrast angiography of the pulmonary veins
D. Contrast angiography of the aorta
E. A 4-chamber cine image obtained at the mid-ventricular level

Correct answer is D.

The likely diagnosis is patent ductus arteriosus, or some other left-to-right communication distal to the level of flow measurements. Among the proposed options, contrast-enhanced angiography of the thoracic aorta is the most likely to demonstrate the correct diagnosis [2, 3]. An intracardiac left-to-right shunt would result in a Qp/Qs > 1, and, thus, atrial–septal defect, ventricular–septal defect, or anomalous pulmonary venous connection would not be likely diagnoses.

3. In the case described in Question 2, which of the following findings would be expected?

A. Dilation of the left ventricle
B. Dilation of the right ventricle
C. Normal size for both left and right ventricles
D. Concentric hypertrophy of the left ventricle
E. Concentric hypertrophy of the right ventricle

Correct answer is A.

Patent ductus arteriosus (and any other extracardiac left-to-right communication) applies extra volume load to the left ventricle that has to circulate both the forward systemic flow and the shunt volume. This results in left ventricular dilation without concentric hypertrophy, similar to any other volume-loading conditions (e.g., aortic regurgitation). Left ventricular dilation also occurs with a ventricular septal defect because the left-to-right shunting occurs primarily during systole and, thus, the right ventricle is usually not particularly affected. Left-to-right shunts at the level of the atria cause right heart dilation because of the increased blood volume with which the right heart is challenged.

4. In a young patient with left-to-right shunt, the following measurements are obtained during a CMR study:

Left ventricular end-diastolic volume: 120 mL
Left ventricular end-systolic volume: 40 mL
Right ventricular end-diastolic volume: 240 mL
Right ventricular end-systolic volume: 100 mL
Aortic root systolic forward flow: 80 mL
Pulmonary trunk systolic forward flow: 120 mL
No aortic or pulmonary valve regurgitation is present.

Which is the most likely diagnosis?

A. Intraventricular septal defect
B. Atrial septal defect
C. Endocardial cushion defect
D. Patent ductus arteriosus
E. Coronary fistula to the right atrium

Correct answer is B.

This patient has a Qp/Qs of 120 mL/80 mL = 1.5, therefore, has a left-to-right shunt that occurs proximal to the point of measurement of blood flow (i.e., the root of the aorta and pulmonary trunk). The left ventricular stroke volume (end-diastolic minus end-systolic volume, i.e., 120 – 40 = 80 mL) is identical to the aortic root systolic forward flow. Therefore, the ventricle does not participate in the shunt. The left-to-right communication occurs before the left ventricle, and, thus, the possible diagnoses would be atrial septal defect or/and anomalous connection of pulmonary veins to the right atrium.

5. The image in Fig. 6.3 is a single frame from a 4-chamber cine study of a young female with persistent atrial arrhythmias.

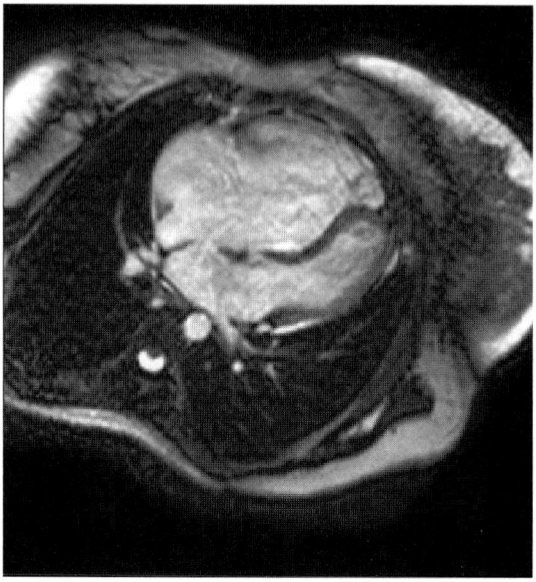

Which is the correct diagnosis?

A. Uhl's cardiomyopathy
B. Arrhythmogenic right ventricular dysplasia
C. Ebstein anomaly
D. Constrictive pericarditis
E. Restrictive cardiomyopathy

The correct answer is C.

Ebstein anomaly is characterized by low attachment of the septal and posterior leaflets of the tricuspid valve (apical displacement of the septal leaflet >8 mm/m^2 compared with the mitral valve annulus). This results in atrialization of a large part of the right ventricle with subsequent marked right atrial enlargement and, clinically, usually presents with various forms of supraventricular arrhythmias. CMR in patients with Ebstein anomaly can establish the diagnosis and evaluate the size and function of the right ventricle [4], measures that are related to patient prognosis and may guide the selection of surgical versus medical management. In the image in Fig. 6.4, the attachment of the tricuspid valve to the mid-apical intraventricular septum is indicated by the long *black arrow*. Ebstein anomaly is almost always associated with an atrial septal defect (*ASD*).

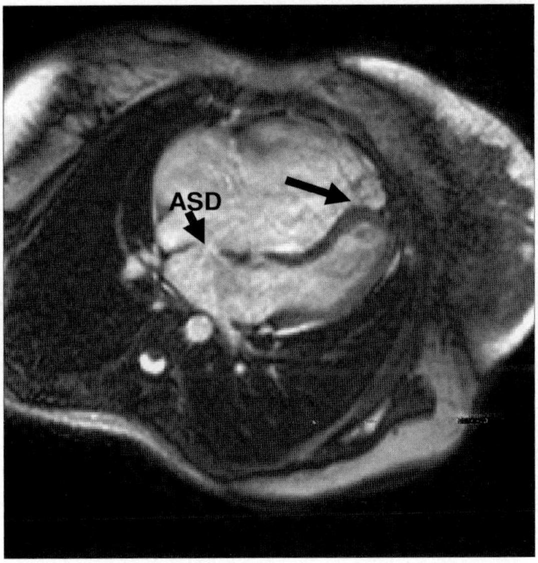

6. The image in Fig. 6.5 is an oblique sagittal black blood image from a CMR study of a young girl with hypertension.

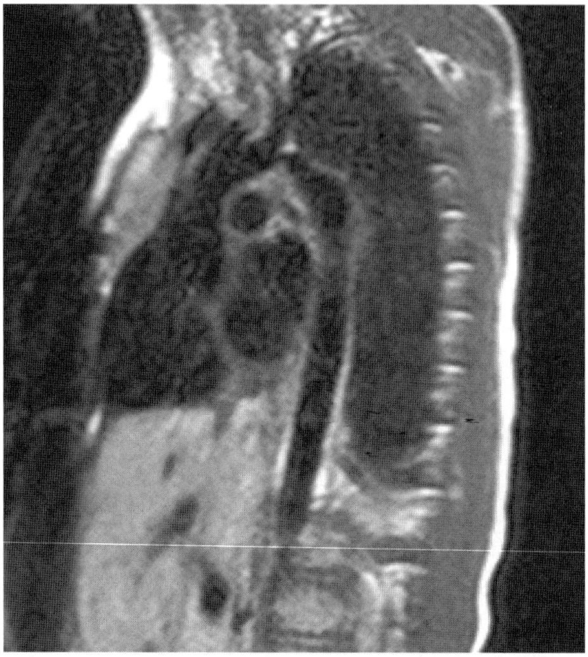

What is the diagnosis?

A. Valvular aortic stenosis
B. Patent ductus arteriosus
C. Coarctation
D. Interruption of the aorta
E. Descending thoracic aortic dissection

The correct answer is C.

The aortic lumen decreases in diameter at the distal arch, immediately after the take-off of the left subclavian artery (*sca*) (Fig. 6.6). Following the site of maximal stenosis (*arrow*), there is poststenotic dilation (*open arrow*). These findings are typical of coarctation. CMR can visualize the anatomy of the entire aorta, assess aortic lumen flow velocities, visualize collateral vessels, and quantify the collateral circulation [5, 6]. Although coarctation can be associated with bicuspid aortic valve, in the image in Fig. 6.6, no comment can be made regarding the presence of valvular aortic stenosis. Interruption of the aorta is an extreme form of coarctation, characterized by discontinuity between ascending and descending thoracic aorta, which is not the case here. There are no findings to suggest descending thoracic aortic dissection (dissection flap or visualization of true and false lumens).

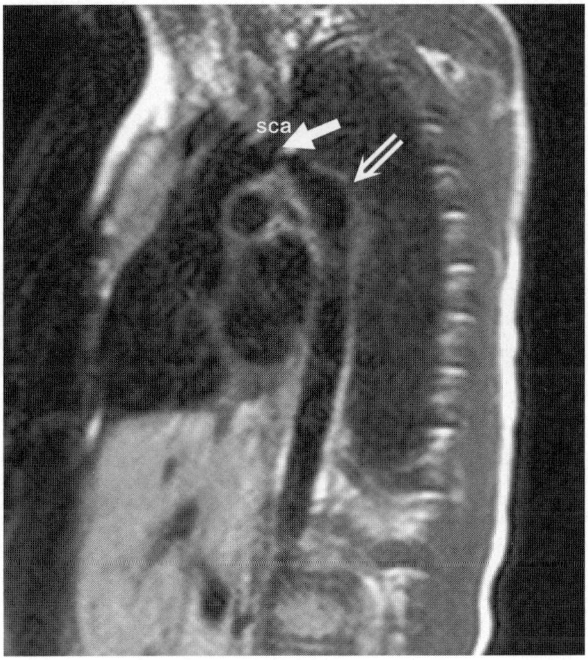

7. Figure 6.7 is a black blood CMR image obtained in the 4-chamber orientation from a young female patient with dyspnea.

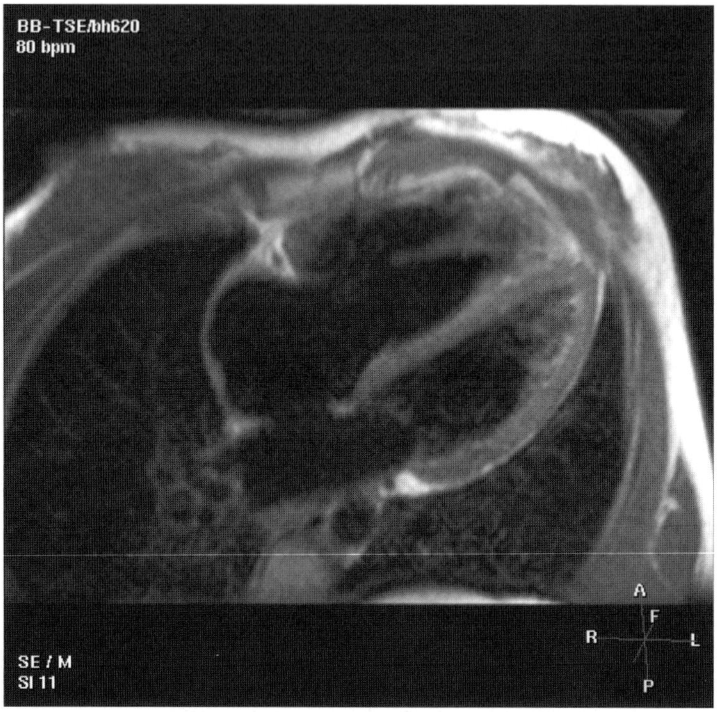

The correct diagnosis is:

A. Ventricular septal defect
B. Atrial septal defect
C. Patent ductus arteriosus
D. Ebstein anomaly
E. Coarctation

Correct answer is B.

The image in Fig. 6.8 demonstrates a dilated right atrium (*ra*) and right ventricle (*RV*), and a discontinuity of the intra-atrial septum (*arrows*). The discontinuity of the intra-atrial septum itself is not diagnostic; signal loss at the septum may be seen with a highly mobile septum and also in thin individuals. However, the dilation of both right atrium and ventricle suggests that the left-to-right communication is likely at the atrial level [7]. Patent ductus arteriosus would result in dilation of the left ventricle. The *dotted line* shows the plane of the tricuspid annulus and the *solid line* shows the plane of the mitral valve annulus, suggesting that the diagnosis of Ebstein anomaly is unlikely. There is no evidence of left ventricular concentric hypertrophy that one would expect with coarctation.

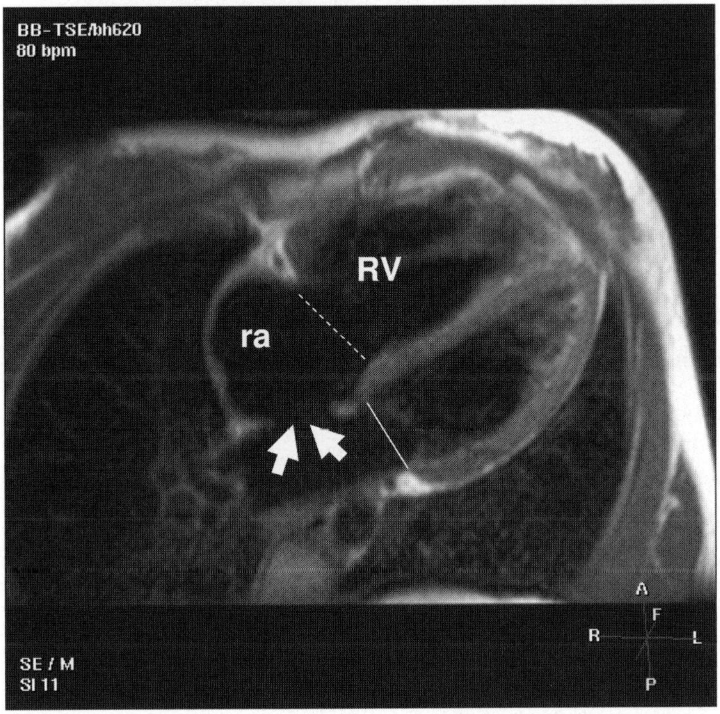

8. The image in Fig. 6.9 is an oblique sagittal image from a dataset of three-dimensional gadolinium-enhanced CMR angiography.

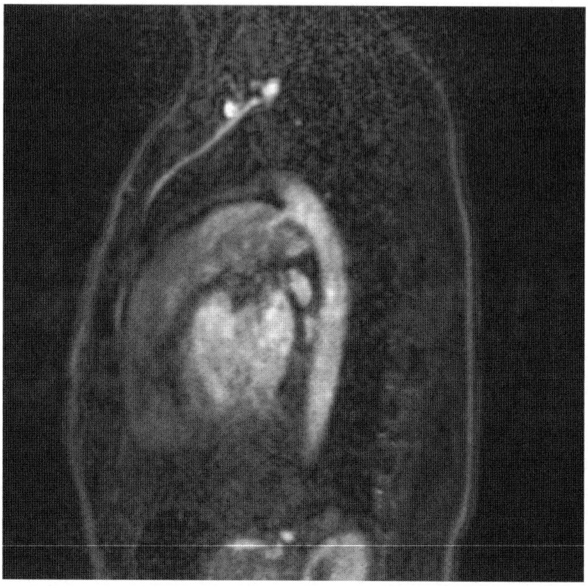

Which is the correct diagnosis?

A. Aortic coarctation
B. Bovine aortic arch
C. Patent ductus arteriosus
D. D-transposition of the great arteries
E. Williams syndrome

Correct answer is C.

In the image in Fig. 6.10, the *arrow* demonstrates the patent ductus arteriosus, connecting the aorta (*ao*) with the pulmonary artery (*pa*). The pulmonary artery is anterior to the aortic root (*ao.r.*), as usual. The arch vessels are not seen in the image in Fig. 6.10, therefore, no comment can be made regarding whether there is bovine arch (common origin of the inanimate and left common carotid). Similarly, the ascending thoracic aorta is not seen, thus, the diagnosis of Williams syndrome cannot be supported by this image. The diameter of the descending aorta distal to the isthmus is normal, eliminating the possibility of aortic coarctation.

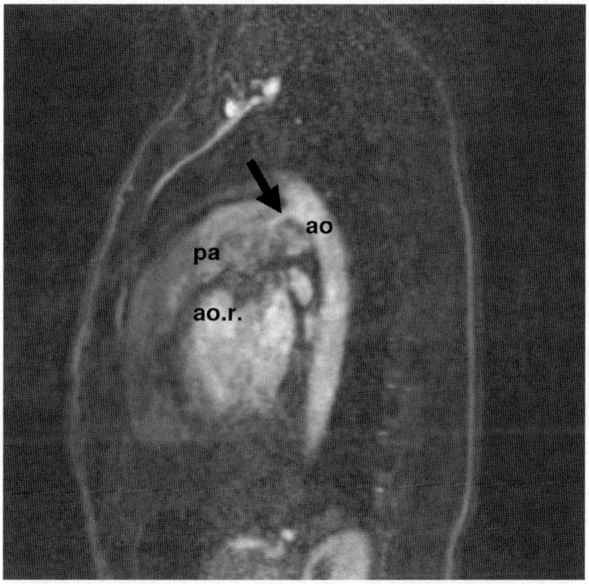

9. A patient with dyspnea is referred for CMR. Transverse black blood images demonstrate dilation of the root of the pulmonary artery. The differential should include all the following *except* for:

A. Pulmonary embolism
B. Atrial septal defect
C. Ventricular septal defect
D. Anomalous return of pulmonary veins to the right atrium
E. Uncorrected tetralogy of Fallot

Correct answer is E.

Pulmonary embolism is frequently associated with pulmonary artery dilation caused by the elevated pressures in the pulmonic circulation. Atrial and ventricular septal defects and anomalous return of the pulmonary veins all result in left-to-right shunt and increase the pulmonic blood flow, which could well account for dilation of the pulmonary artery. Tetralogy of Fallot is characterized by a stenotic and frequently hypoplastic pulmonary artery. In patients with corrected tetralogy of Fallot, dilation of the root of the pulmonary artery may be frequently seen, depending on the surgical correction method and the insufficiency of the pulmonic valve.

10. The image in Fig. 6.11 is a reformatted image from a high-resolution white blood CMR study obtained during ventricular diastole at the base of the heart in a young patient with congenital heart disease.

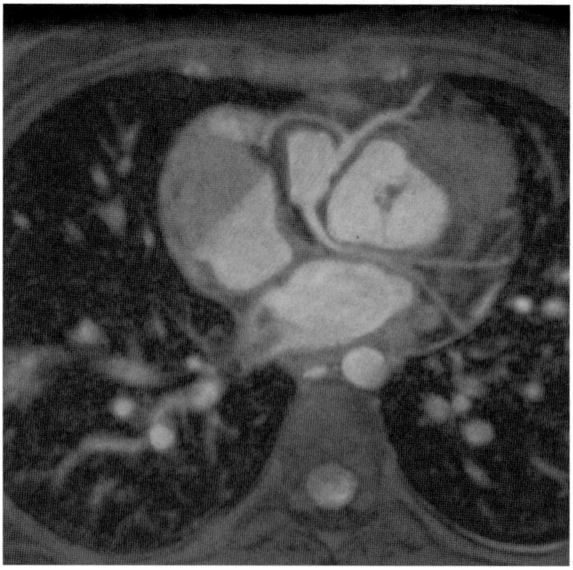

Which of the following abnormalities is *not* demonstrated by the image?

A. Transposition of the great arteries
B. Pulmonary valve insufficiency
C. Anomalous takeoff of the coronary arteries
D. Dilation of the pulmonary artery
E. Anomalous pulmonary venous return

Correct answer is E.

The aorta (*Ao*) is anterior to the pulmonary artery (*PA*), consistent with the diagnosis of transposition of the great arteries (*TGA*) (Fig. 6.12) [8]. The pulmonary artery root has a much larger diameter than the aorta, consistent with pulmonary artery dilation. At the coaptation of the cusps of the pulmonic valve (*black arrow*), there is signal void, consistent with central pulmonary regurgitation. There are two coronary arteries (*white arrows*) originating from the aortic root that have a non-typical course (in fact, this course is characteristic of patients with transposition of the great arteries).

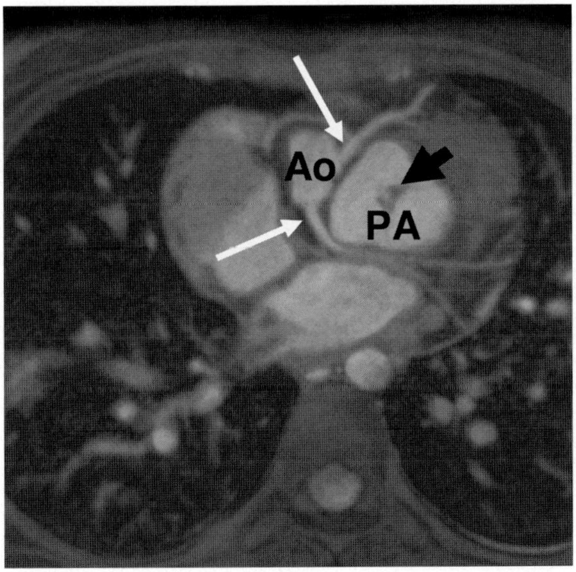

11. In patients with tetralogy of Fallot who have undergone total surgical correction, which of the following is *not* an expected finding on follow-up CMR evaluation several years later?

A. Dilation of the right ventricle
B. Insufficiency of the pulmonic valve
C. Supravalvular aortic stenosis
D. Borderline or normal left ventricular systolic function
E. Regional wall motion abnormality at the right ventricular outflow tract

Correct answer is C.

After surgical correction of tetralogy of Fallot, there is usually wall motion abnormality at the right ventricular outflow tract, at the site of the free wall ventriculotomy and patch placement. There is also usually some deformation of the pulmonary valve apparatus, resulting in pulmonary regurgitation. In fact, patients frequently need to be reoperated for pulmonary valve insufficiency several years after the initial correction. Some degree of right ventricular dilation is almost always seen, whereas the left ventricle usually has borderline systolic function. Among patients with tetralogy of Fallot, many have aortic root dilation. Supravalvular aortic stenosis is not an expected finding. CMR is a valuable modality for sequential follow-up examinations in patients with surgically corrected tetralogy of Fallot [9].

12. The image in Fig. 6.13 is a coronal localizer obtained in a 15-year-old patient who was referred for CMR for evaluation of congenital heart disease.

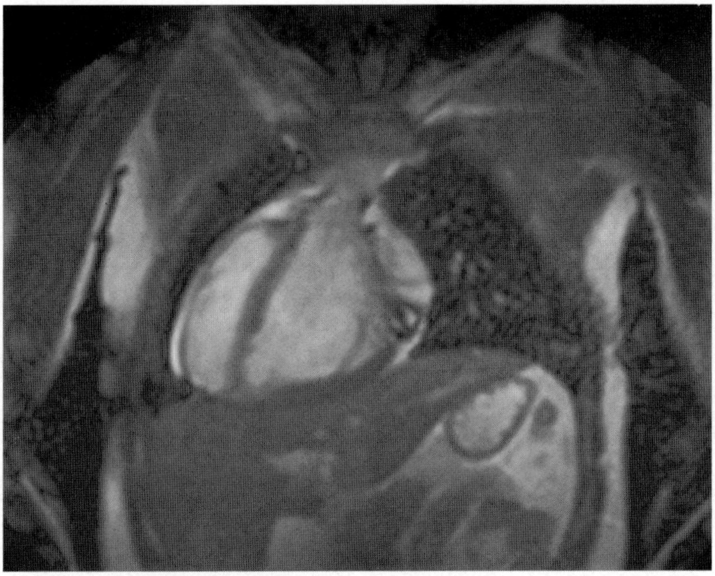

Which is the correct diagnosis?

A. Levocardia, situs inversus
B. Mesocardia, situs solitus
C. Mesocardia, situs inversus
D. Dextrocardia, situs solitus
E. Dextrocardia, situs inversus

Correct answer is D.

Levocardia refers to the heart being located at the left hemithorax. Mesocardia (from the Greek word mesi, middle) refers to a middle position of the heart inside the chest cavity, and dextrocardia suggest that the heart is located in the right hemithorax. Situs solitus suggests a normal location of the abdominal viscera, whereas situs inversus is the term used to describe the mirror image of the abdominal contents. In Fig. 6.13, the heart is in the right hemithorax (dextrocardia) and the liver is also on the right (situs solitus).

13. The patient that was discussed in the Question 12 (dextrocardia, situs solitus) also underwent a gadolinium-enhanced CMR angiogram. The images in Fig. 6.14 were all obtained in the coronal orientation, with A to D progressing from anterior to posterior.

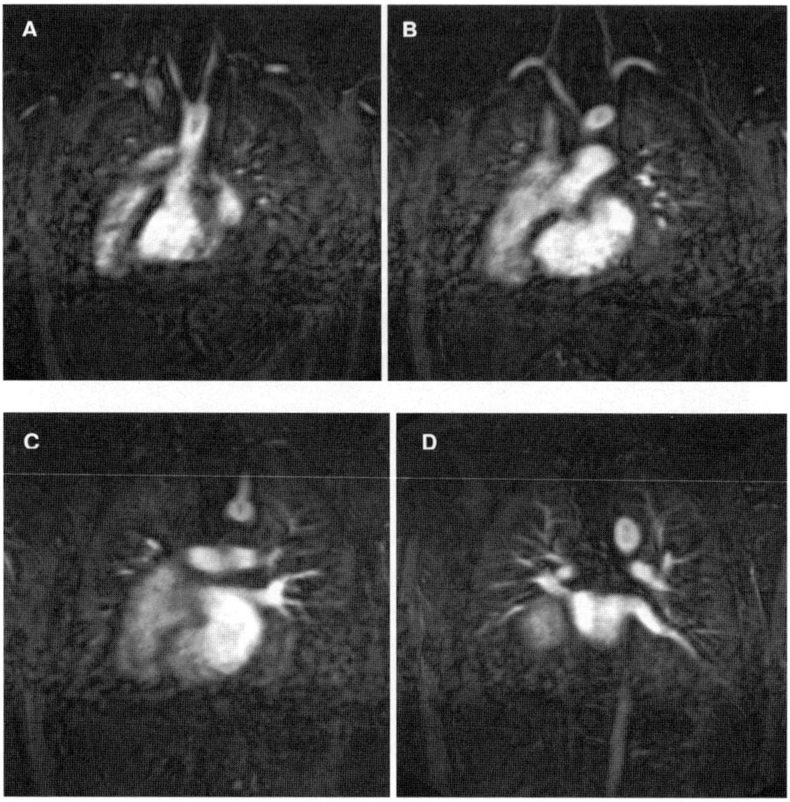

In addition to dextrocardia, situs solitus, what is the correct diagnosis?

A. Total anomalous pulmonary venous return
B. Tetralogy of Fallot
C. Congenitally corrected transposition of the great arteries
D. No other cardiac abnormalities
E. Coarctation

Correct answer is C.

In the images in Fig. 6.15, the cardiac structures are labeled (*AA*, aortic arch; *AAo*, ascending aorta; *DAo*, descending thoracic aorta; *LA*, left atrium; *LPA*, left pulmonary artery; *LLPV*, left lower pulmonary vein; *LUPV*, left upper pulmonary vein; *PA*, pulmonary artery; *RPA*, right pulmonary artery; *RUPV*, right upper pulmonary vein; *SVC*, superior vena cava). The aortic root is anterior to the pulmonary artery trunk, consistent with transposition of the great arteries. The pulmonary veins return normally to the left atrium that connects to the systemic ventricle (atrioventricular discordance), which appears to have right ventricular characteristics (different inflow–outflow), thereby establishing the diagnosis of congenitally corrected transposition of the great arteries [10]. The other characteristics that suggest an anatomical right systemic ventricle (moderator band, increased trabeculations, and connection to a tricuspid valve) are not readily evident from these images, although they were all present in this patient.

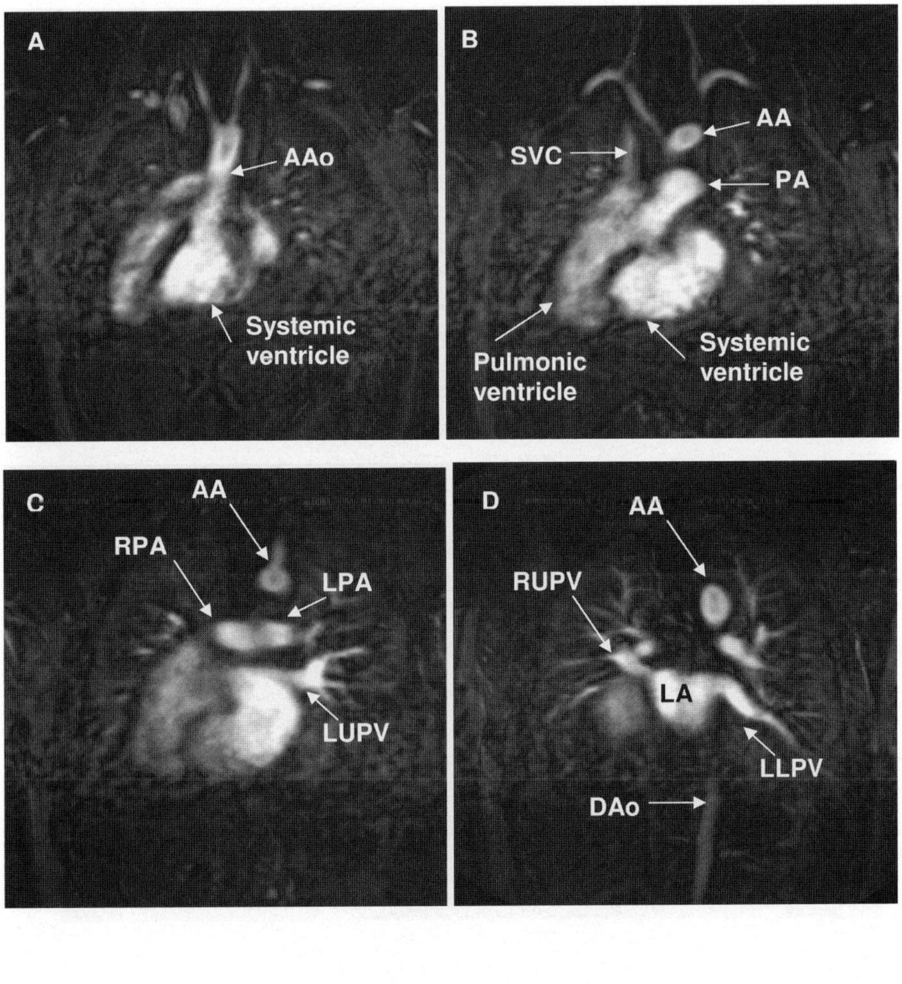

14. A middle-aged woman is referred for a CMR study for evaluation of possible intracardiac shunt. Phase-contrast images are obtained at the proximal aorta and pulmonary artery, and the analysis of these images is presented in the Fig. 6.16 (A, aorta; B, pulmonary artery [facing page]).

Based on the results of this study, you would conclude that:

A. There is an intracardiac left-to-right shunt with Qp/Qs >2
B. There is an extracardiac left-to-right shunt (probably caused by a patent ductus arteriosus) with a Qp/Qs >2
C. There is an extracardiac left-to-right shunt (probably caused by a patent ductus arteriosus) with a Qp/Qs <0.5
D. There is no evidence for a left-to-ight or right-to-left shunt
E. There is evidence for intracardiac right-to-left shunt with Qp/Qs <0.5

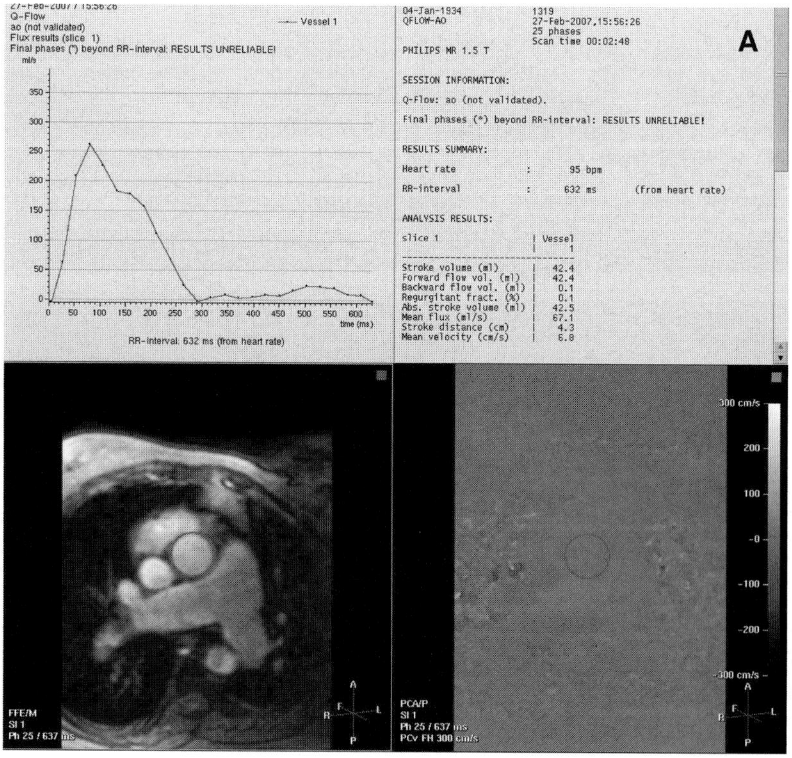

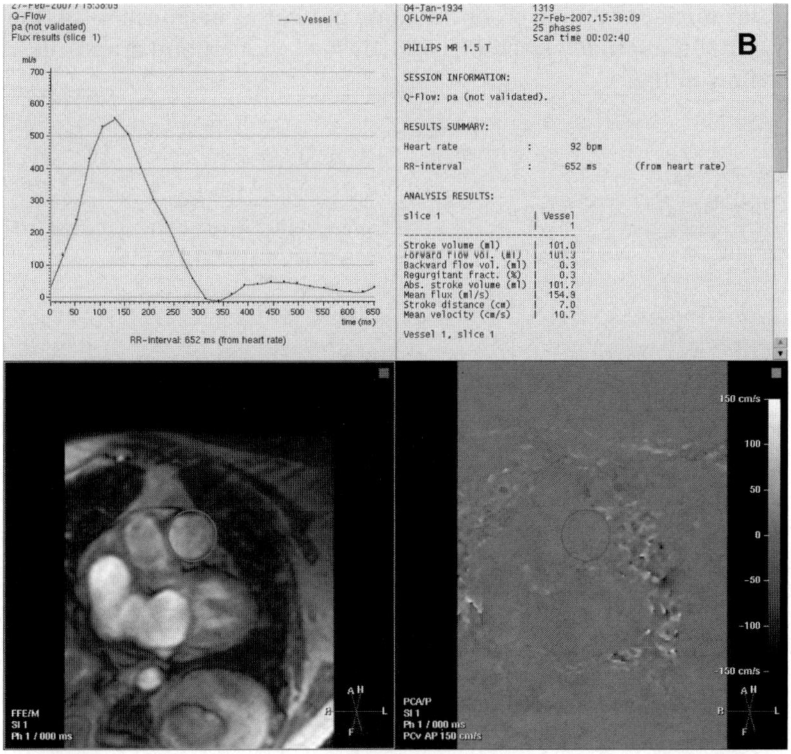

Correct answer is A.

The flow analysis demonstrates an aortic forward flow of 42 ml (Fig. 6.16A) and a pulmonic forward flow of 101 ml (Fig. 6.16B). Therefore, the ratio Qp/Qs is 101/42 = 2.4. This suggests the presence of an intracardiac left to right shunt. An intracardiac right-to-left shunt would provide Qp<Qs, because the systemic circulation would be accommodating greater volumes (the pulmonic forward flow plus the shunt flow). The same would happen with an extracardiac shunt at the level of the great arteries (i.e., patent ductus arteriosus), in which the Qp would be smaller than the Qs. From the data presented here, one cannot be certain about the site of communication (i.e., atria versus ventricles versus both).

15. In the aortic flow analysis of the same patient as in Question 14, the flow profile of the second vessel (Fig. 6.17, dashed contour and graph), describes the flow in the:

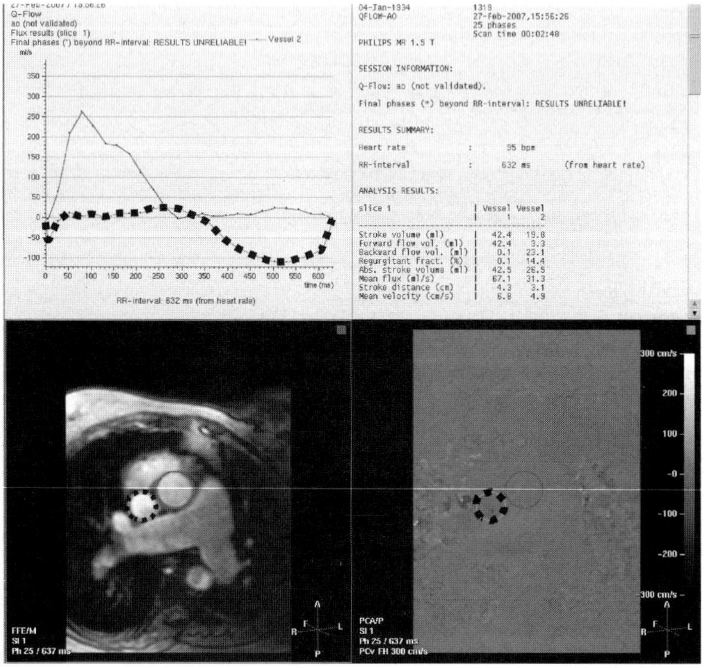

A. Pulmonary artery
B. Superior vena cava
C. Inferior vena cava
D. Right pulmonary artery
E. Left pulmonary artery

Correct answer is B.

The normal location of the superior vena cava is to the right and slightly posterior to the ascending aorta. The flow in the vena cavae is occurring during ventricular diastole and has opposite direction to that of the ascending aorta. The total flow in the superior vena cava is normally approximately one third of the total cardiac output. All of these findings are evident in the *dashed* graph in Fig. 6.17.

16. A young adult with cyanotic congenital heart disease is referred for CMR to assess cardiovascular anatomy and function. At an early age, the patient underwent a modified Blalock–Taussig shunt. In Figure 6.18, A is a single transverse slice from a black blood study; B is a maximal intensity projection (MIP) of the contrast-enhanced CMR angiography; and C and D are diastolic and systolic transverse slices at the base of the heart.

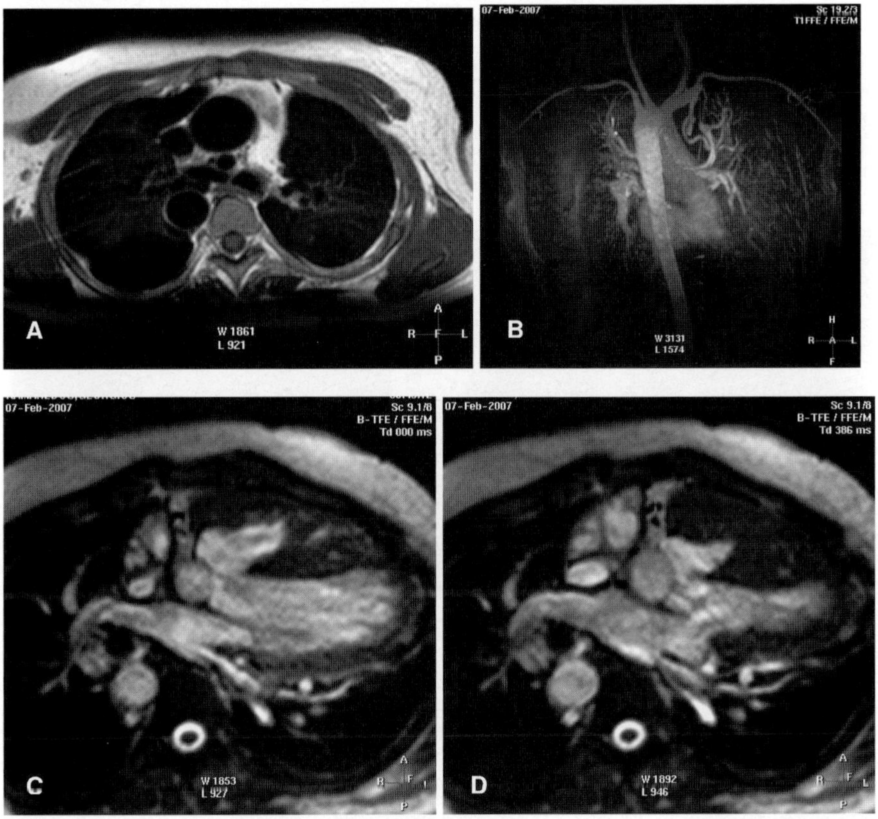

What is the most likely diagnosis for this patient?

A. Common variant of tetralogy of Fallot
B. Truncus arteriosus
C. Transposition of the great arteries
D. Interruption of the aortic arch
E. Tricuspid atresia

Correct answer is B.

In Fig. 6.19, *A* demonstrates the location of the ascending aorta (*AAo*), superior vena cava (*SVC*), and descending thoracic aorta (*DAo*). The right and left main stem bronchi are also indicated (*RB* and *LB*, respectively). The aorta crosses the right main stem bronchus, thus, forming a right arch. *B* shows the systemic-to-pulmonic communications, which include the modified B–T shunt (*white dotted arrow*) and aortopulmonary collaterals (*white solid arrows*). *C* and *D* demonstrate the large ventricular septal defect (*VSD*) connecting the right and left ventricles (*RV* and *VL*, respectively). The aortic valve (*AV*) overrides the ventricular septal defect, but there is no pulmonary artery present. These findings are typical for truncus arteriosus type IV. Extreme variant of tetralogy of Fallot (also named pseudotruncus) with atresia of the pulmonary artery may also have a similar appearance [11].

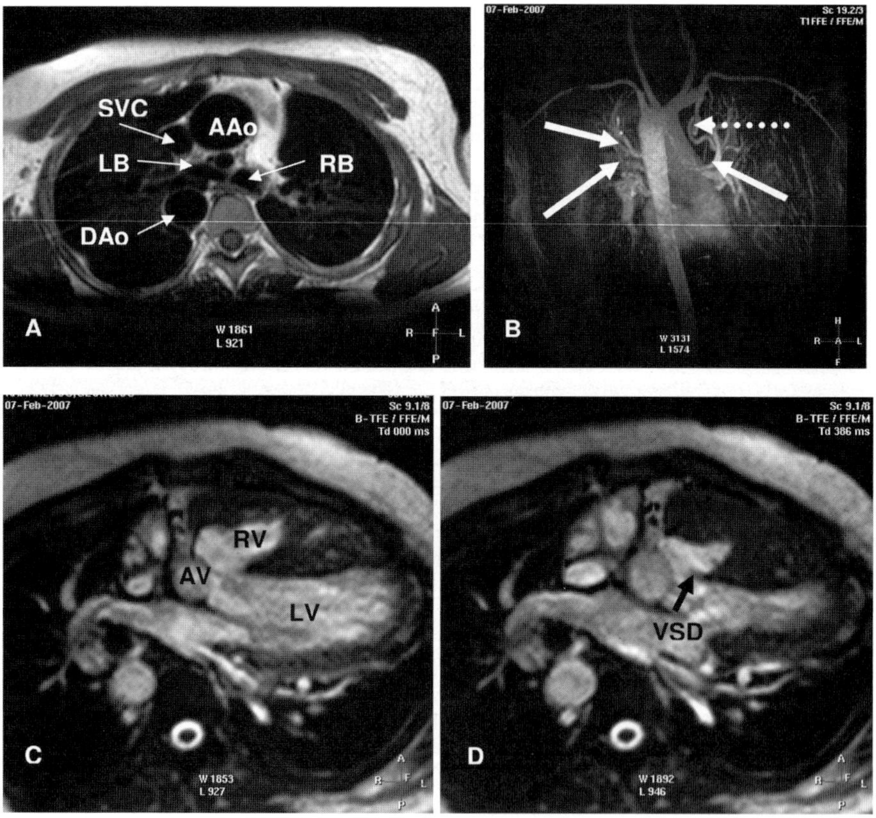

17. A young adult is referred for a CMR study because of an abnormal echocardiogram obtained during evaluation of palpitations. The anatomic transverse T1-weighted images at three levels are displayed in Fig. 6.20 (A, more cranial; C, more caudal).

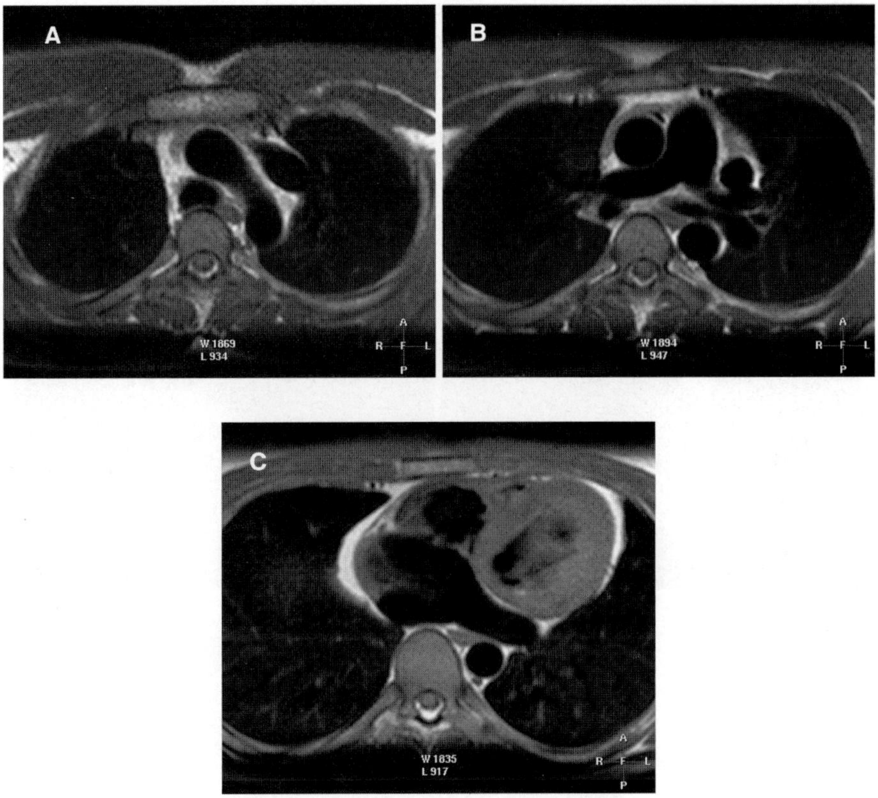

What is the diagnosis?

A. Atrial septal defect
B. Transposition of the great arteries
C. Anomalous pulmonary venous return
D. Ebstein anomaly
E. Persistent left superior vena cava

Correct answer is E.

The anatomic structures, including the ascending aorta (*AAo*), aortic arch (*arch*), descending thoracic aorta (*DAo*), coronary sinus (*CS*), persistent left superior vena cava (*LSVC*), right atrium (*RA*), and trachea (*T*), are labeled in Fig. 6.21. *A* demonstrates the absence of right superior vena cava, which should be at the right of the aorta [12]. The pulmonary artery is not dilated (approximately the same size as the aorta), arguing against left-to-right communication (caused by atrial septal defect, anomalous pulmonary venous return, ventricular septal defect, etc.). The attachment of the tricuspid valve to the intraventricular septum in *C* appears to be normal, arguing against Ebstein's anomaly.

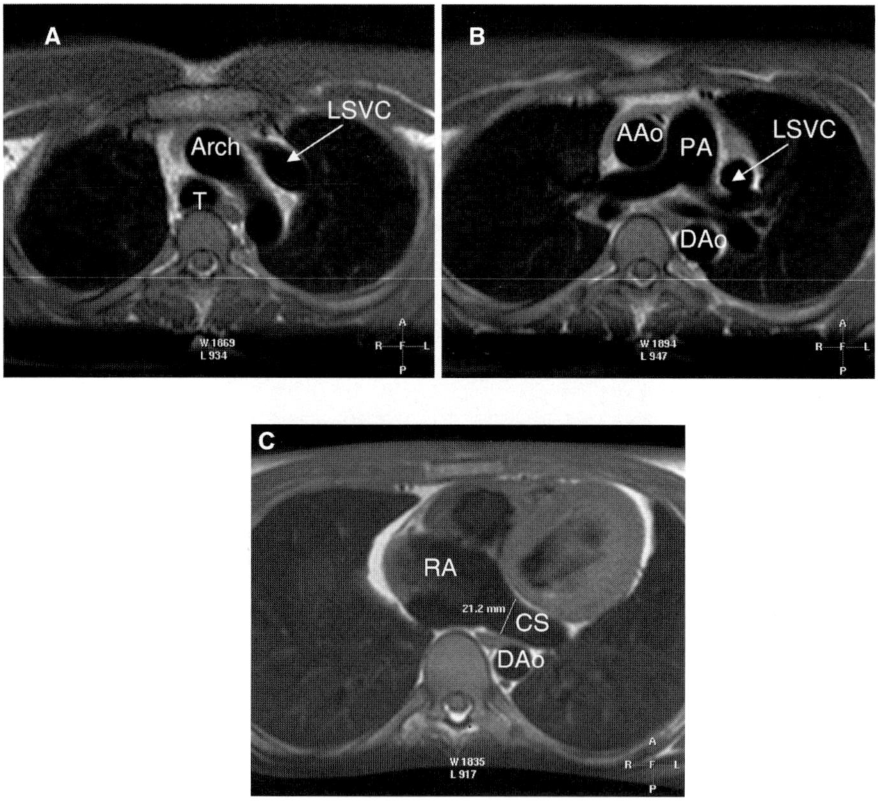

18. A middle-aged woman presented with supraventricular arrhythmias and palpitations. The echocardiogram suggested the diagnosis, but, for precise anatomic and functional assessment, a CMR study was requested. The images in Fig. 6.22 are diastolic (A) and systolic (B) black blood images of the heart in the transverse orientation.

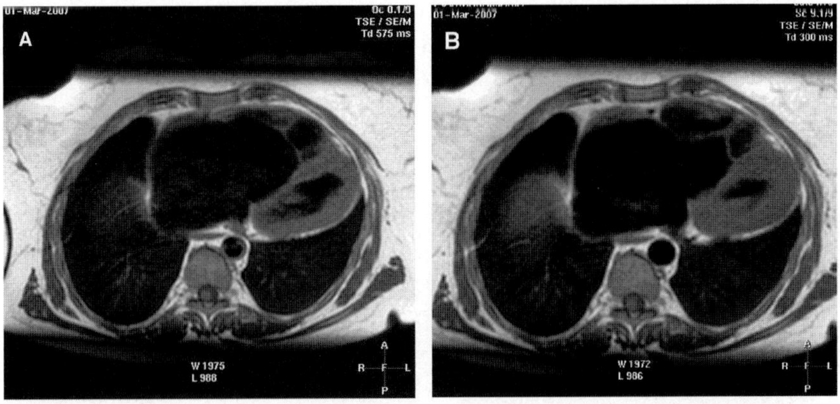

What is the diagnosis?

A. Tricuspid valve atresia
B. Pulmonary valve atresia
C. Hypoplastic left ventricle
D. Single ventricle
E. Ebstein anomaly

Correct answer is E.

The images in Fig. 6.23 demonstrate a low attachment of the septal leaflet of the tricuspid valve (*A white arrow*). The right atrium (*RA*), right ventricle (*RV*), coronary sinus (*CS*), and left ventricle (*LV*) are indicated. The precise distance of the tricuspid valve septal attachment from the mitral valve annulus is critical in deciding whether the patient can be surgically corrected or not. Tricuspid atresia is also characterized by a huge right atrium and hypoplastic right ventricle, but the attachment of the atretic tricuspid valve on the intraventricular septum is normal. Pulmonary valve atresia is associated with dilation of both the right atrium and ventricle. In this case, the right ventricle and left ventricle are discrete, and the left ventricle is normal in size.

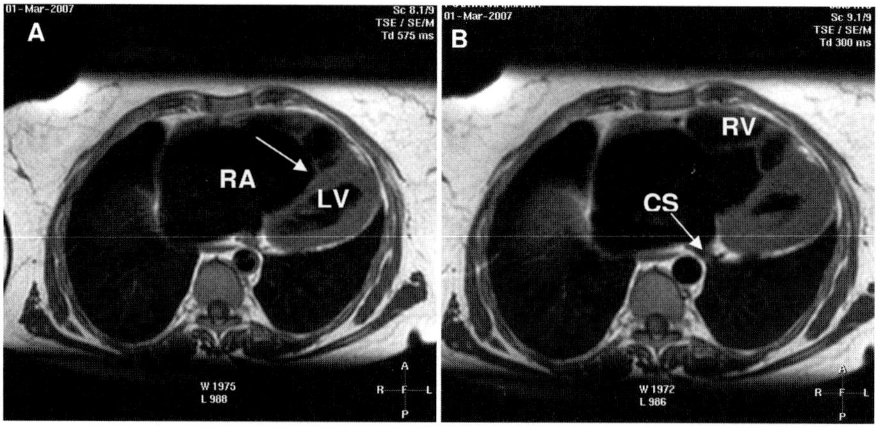

19. Figure 6.24 shows diastolic (A) and systolic (B) images in the short-axis orientation at the base of the heart, and diastolic (C) and systolic (D) images in the 4-chamber orientation.

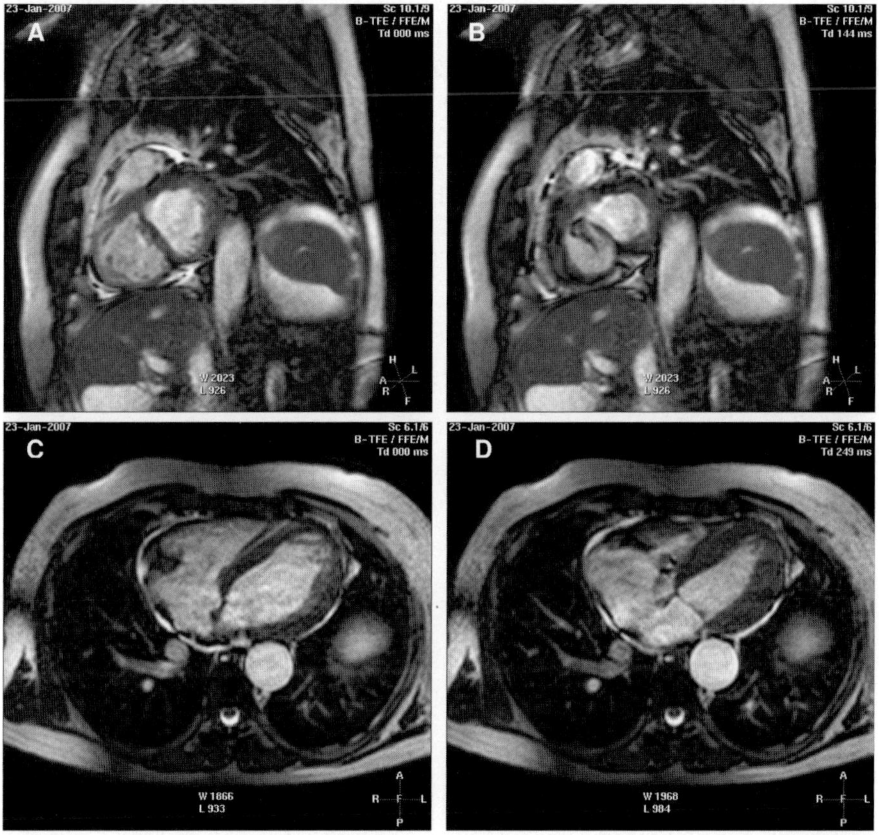

What is the likely diagnosis?

A. Hypertrophic cardiomyopathy
B. Ischemic cardiomyopathy
C. Atrial septal defect
D. Ventricular septal defect
E. Endocardial cushion defect

Correct answer is D.

The systolic images in Fig. 6.25 demonstrate a signal void in the basal portion of the right ventricle, emanating from the basal intraventricular septum (*white arrows*). The size of the defect cannot be precisely assessed by these images. However, the relatively small size of the left ventricle suggests that this is not a hemodynamically significant left-to-right communication. The wall thickness of all walls is similar, arguing against hypertrophic cardiomyoapthy, and systolic function seems to be normal, arguing against ischemic cardiomyopathy. The signal dropout at the intraatrial septum (*D, small black arrow*) is commonly seen in cine images and should not be interpreted as atrial septal defect. There is no other evidence of atrial septal defect or endocardial cushion defect in these images. Although the diagnosis of a ventricular septal defect is usually made by echocardiography, CMR may offer additional precise quantification of the ventricular size and function and Qp/Qs ratio [3, 13, 14].

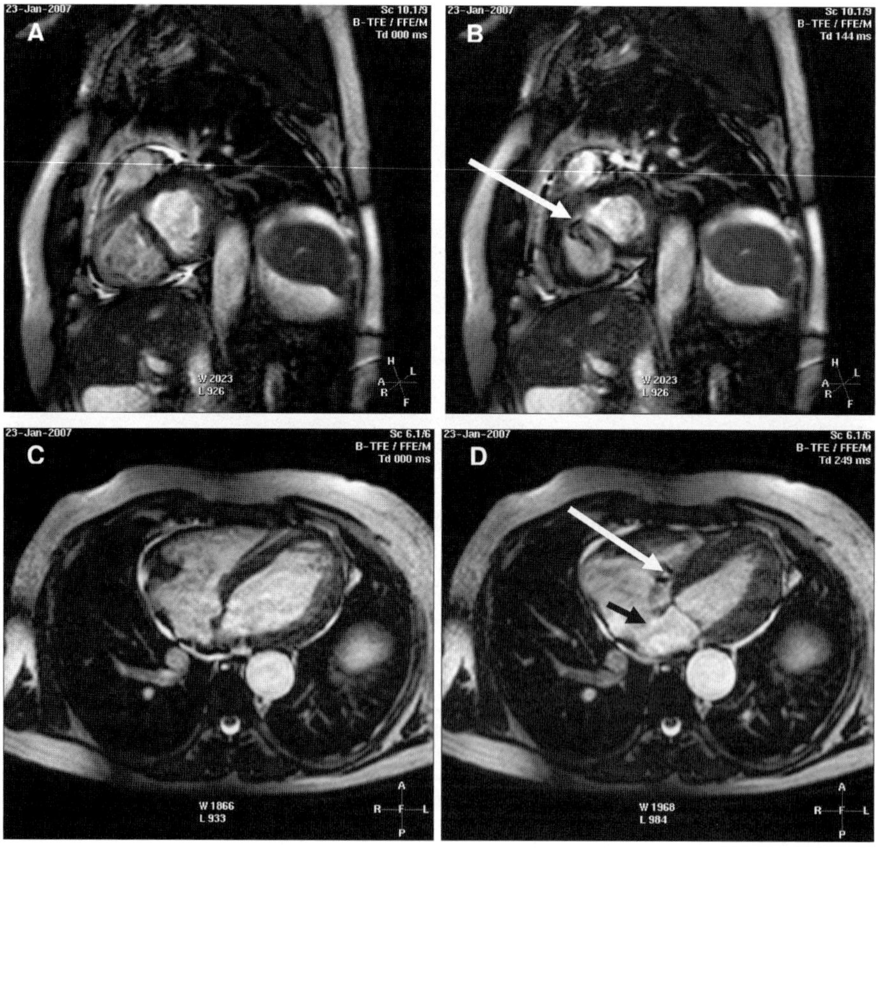

20. The black blood CMR image in Fig. 6.26 was obtained from a patient with known congenital heart disease.

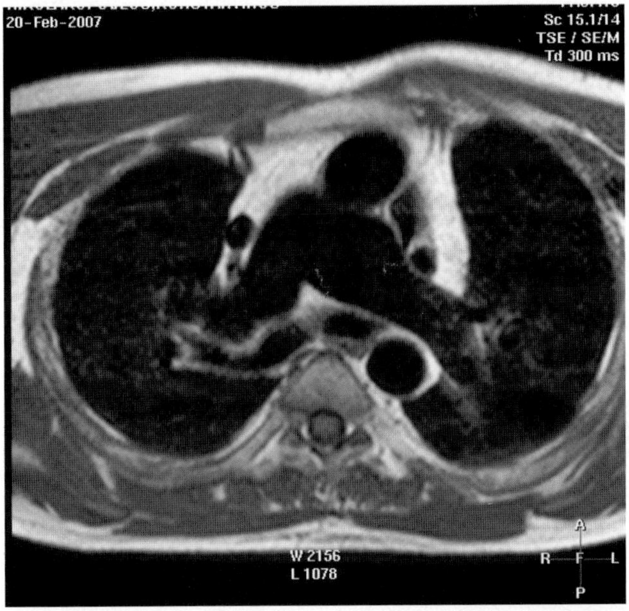

Which of the following entities is *not* demonstrated by the image?

A. Transposition of the great arteries
B. Right aortic arch
C. Persistent left superior vena cava
D. Left aortic arch
E. Dilation of the pulmonary artery

Correct answer is B.

The anatomic structures are labeled in Fig. 6.27 (*AAo*, ascending aorta; *DAo*, descending thoracic aorta; *LMSB*, left main stem bronchus; *LPA*, left pulmonary artery; *LSVC*, left superior vena cava; *PA*, pulmonary artery; *RMSB*, right main stem bronchus; *RPA*, right pulmonary artery; *SVC*, superior vena cava). The ascending aorta is anterior to the pulmonary artery, consistent with transposition of the great arteries. The pulmonary artery and its main branches are dilated. The aorta crosses the left main stem bronchus, thus, giving a left aortic arch. Both the right and left superior vena cava are present.

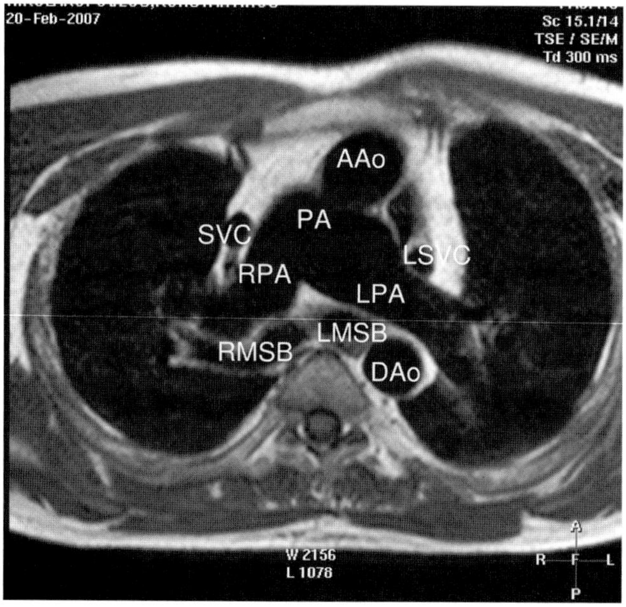

21. The CMR images in Fig. 6.28 were obtained from a young girl with stridor. A and B are bright blood high-resolution images at two levels at the thoracic cavity apex. C is a MIP of the three-dimensional contrast-enhanced CMR angiography.

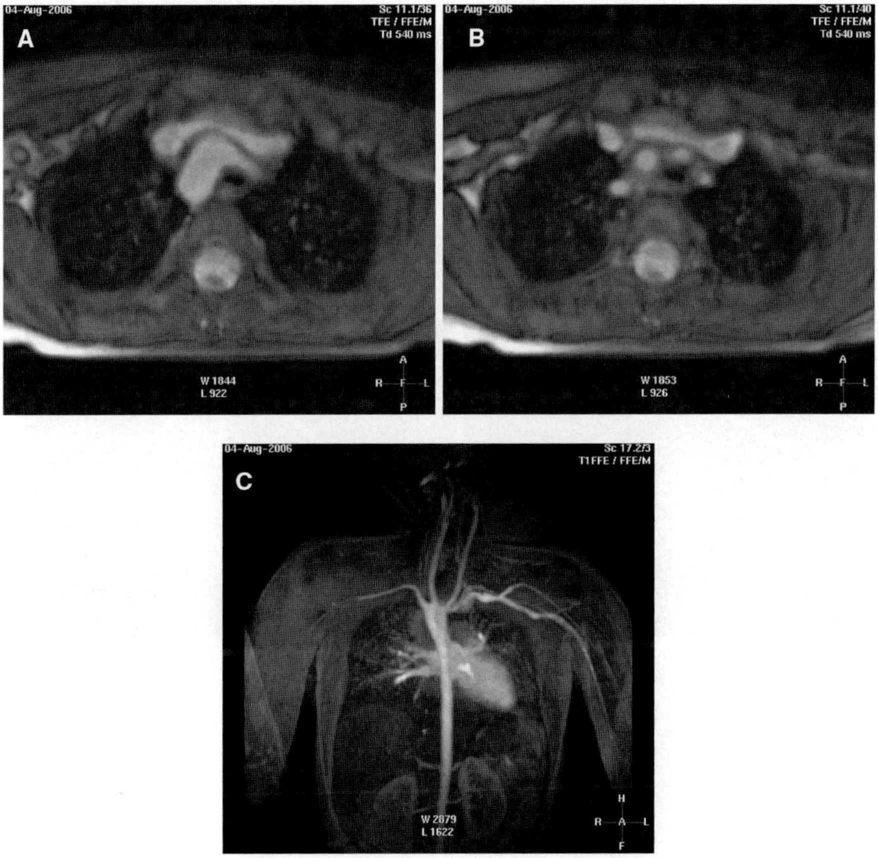

What is the diagnosis?

A. Coarctation
B. Pulmonary sling
C. Right-sided aorta
D. Incomplete aortic ring
E. Williams syndrome

Correct answer is D.

In the images in Fig. 6.29, the right aortic arch (*RAA*) and hypoplastic left aortic arch (*LAA*) are indicated surrounding the trachea (*T*) from the front. The right common carotid (*RCCA*) and right subclavian artery (*RSCLVA*) originate from the right aortic arch, whereas the left common carotid (*LCCA*) and left subclavian artery (*LSCLVA*) originate from the left aortic arch. This is the most common type of aortic ring, accounting for approximately 80% of cases with this congenital vascular abnormality. In those patients in whom both left and right aortic arches persist and join to form the descending thoracic aorta, the trachea and esophagus are enclosed in a complete vascular ring and frequently compressed, with dyspnea with stridor and dysphagia from an early age [15].

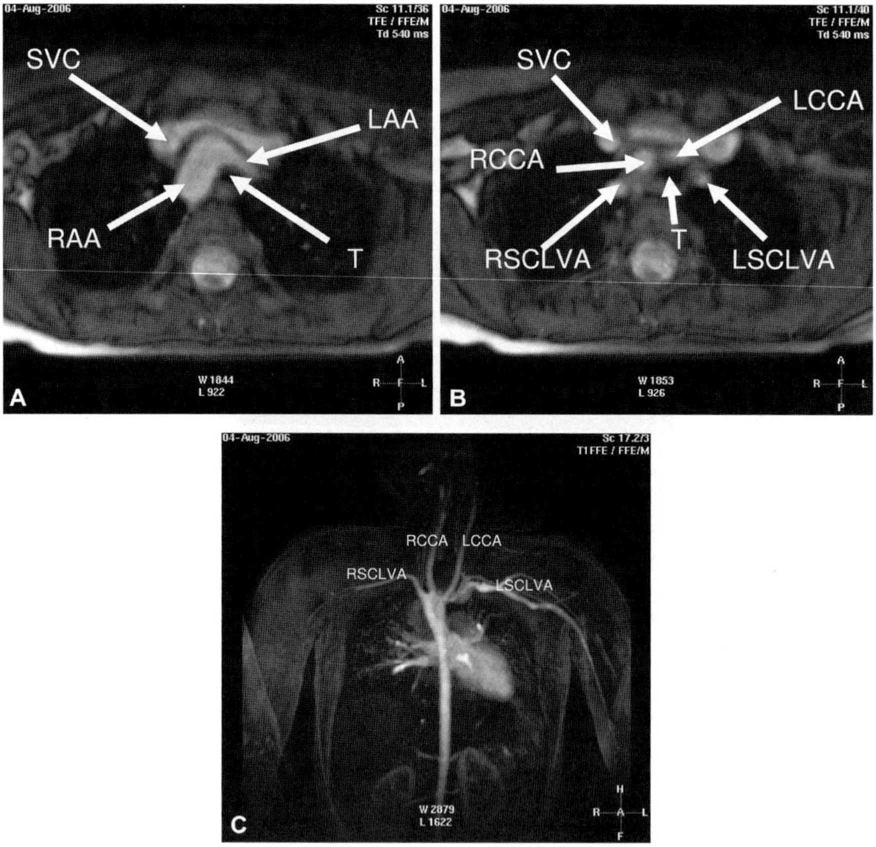

22. A middle-aged man was referred for a CMR study after a failed attempt to cardiac catheterization via the Judkins (femoral) approach for suspected coronary artery disease. The patient did not have a history of hypertension. The image in Fig. 6.30 is a single frame from the three-dimensional contrast-enhanced CMR angiogram.

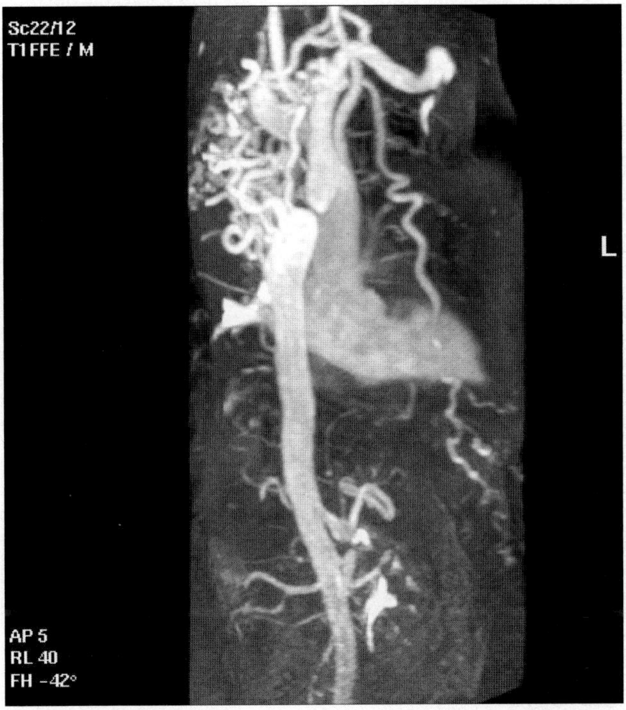

What is the diagnosis?

A. Double aortic arch
B. Coarctation
C. Aortic interruption
D. Takayasu disease
E. Aortic dissection

Correct answer is C.

Aortic interruption is the extreme form of coarctation, in which there is no continuity between the aortic arch and the descending thoracic aorta. The site of interruption in this case is indicated by the *black arrow* in Fig. 6.31. This patient has a highly developed collateral circulation through the intercostal (*white arrows*) and internal mammary (*arrowheads*) arteries, and this is the reason why he did not develop hypertension. There is no evidence of double aortic arch, aortitis, or aortic dissection.

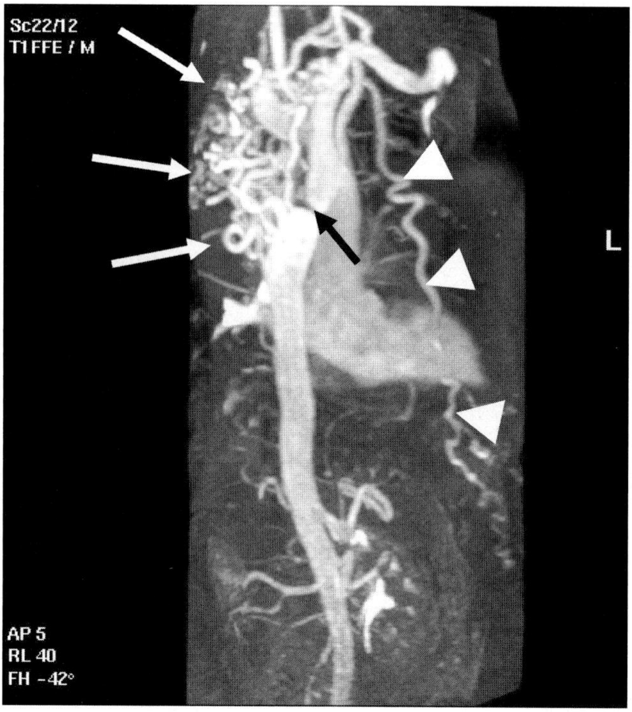

23. The image in Fig. 6.32 is a single slice from a CMR coronary angiogram in a double-oblique orientation along the right atrioventricular groove.

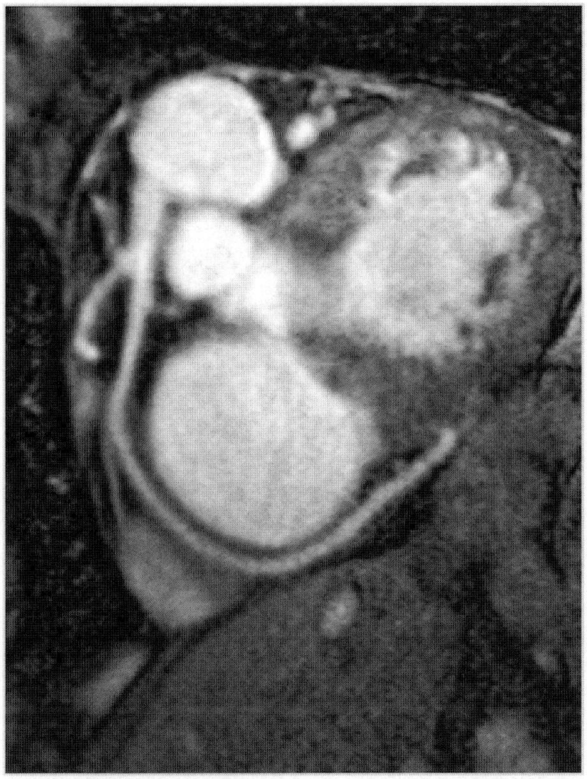

What is the diagnosis?

A. Tight left main stenosis
B. Normal coronary artery anatomy
C. Anomalous takeoff of the right coronary artery from the left sinus of Valsalva
D. Anomalous takeoff of the right coronary from the pulmonary artery
E. Anomalous takeoff of the left main from the right sinus of Valsalva

Correct answer is D.

The aorta (*Ao*), left ventricle (*LV*), pulmonary artery (*PA*), right atrium (*RA*), and right coronary artery (*RCA*) are indicated in Fig. 6.33. The right coronary artery originates from the pulmonary artery instead of the aorta. The right coronary artery diameter is enlarged because the vessel effectively functions as a shunt between the aorta and the pulmonary artery, via highly developed left-to-right coronary artery collaterals (not shown in this image). The flow in this right coronary artery is, thus, retrograde (aorta-to-pulmonary artery).

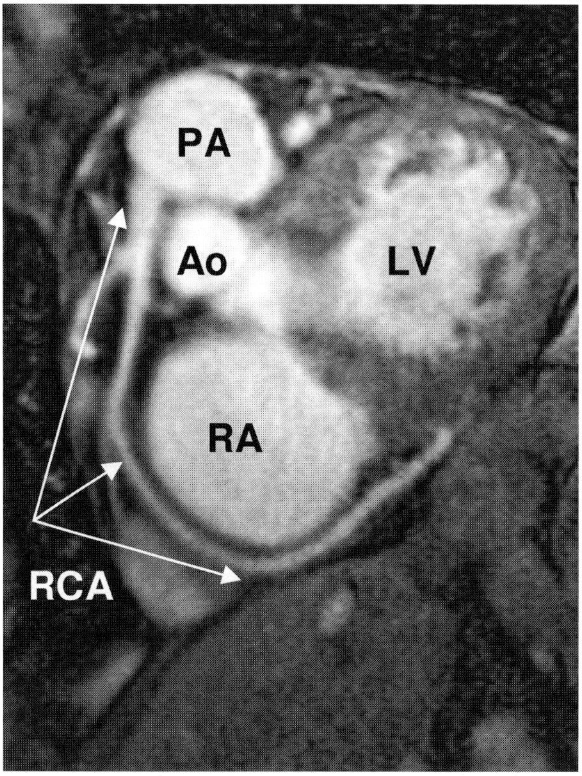

24. A young adult with a history of congenital heart disease is referred for a CMR study years after surgical correction. The images in Fig. 6.34 are transverse bright blood images at several levels (A to D, cranial to caudal).

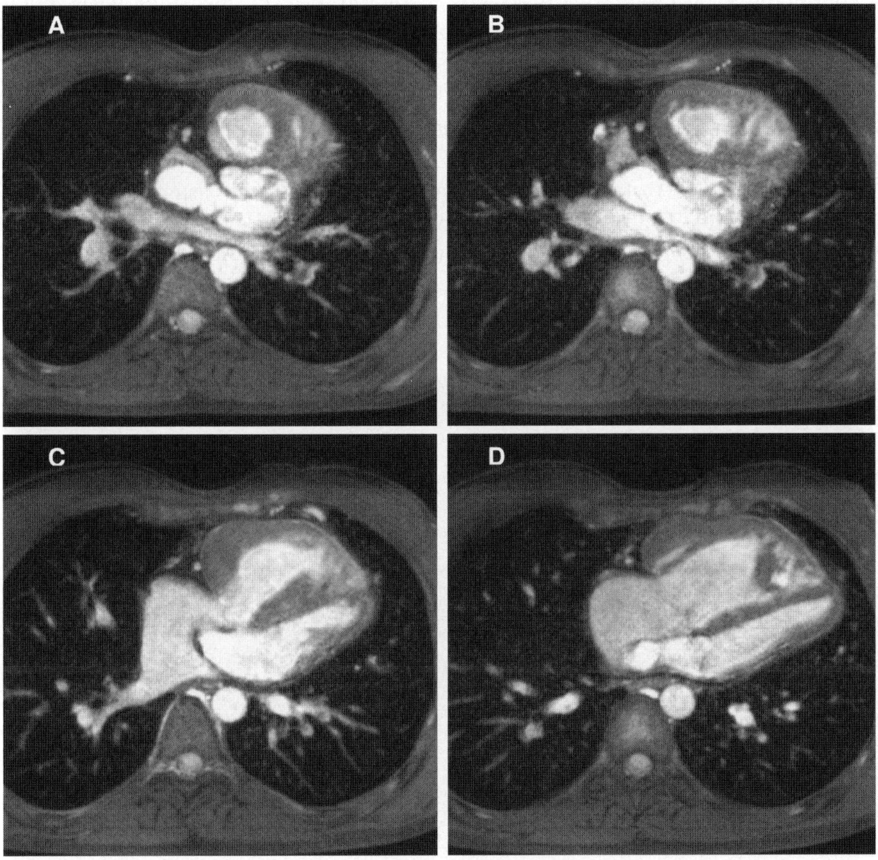

What is the patient's disease and what correction has been performed?

A. Tetralogy of Fallot, total surgical correction
B. Tricuspid atresia, Fontan operation
C. Pulmonary stenosis, Glenn procedure
D. Transposition of the great arteries, atrial switch
E. Transposition of the great arteries, arterial switch

Correct answer is D.

This patient has transposition of the great arteries and has undergone an atrial switch operation, in which the systemic venous return through the superior and inferior vena cava (*SVC* and *IVC*, respectively) is directed to the anatomically left subpulmonic ventricle (*LV*) (Fig. 6.35). At the atrial level, the pulmonary venous blood is directed into the right atrium (*RA*) through a surgically created baffle (*B*). The right atrium connects to the right ventricle (*RV*), which is hypertrophied because it functions as the systemic ventricle. In this particular patient, there is a stenosis of the single left pulmonary vein (*black arrow*) as it crosses between the atrial baffle and the descending thoracic aorta. *Ao*, aorta; *DAo*, descending aorta; *LA*, left atrium; *LPV*, left pulmonary vein; *PA*, pulmonary artery; *RVOT*, right ventricular outflow tract; *RLPV*, right lower pulmonary vein; *RUPV*, right upper pulmonary vein. CMR is uniquely suited to assess patients with complex congenital heart disease before and after surgical correction, such as patients with transposition of the great arteries after atrial switch operations [16].

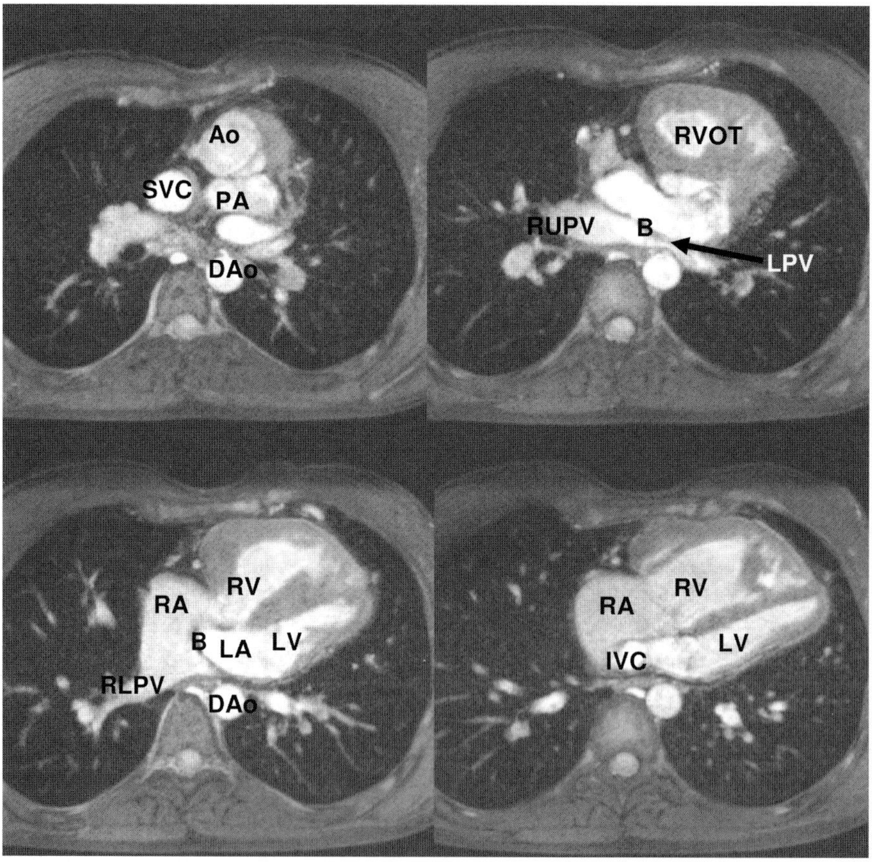

References

1. Danias PG, Stuber M, McConnell MV, and Manning WJ. The diagnosis of congenital coronary anomalies with magnetic resonance imaging. *Coron Artery Dis*, 2001;12(8):621–626.
2. Gaba RC, Carlos RC, Weadock WJ, Reddy GP, Sneider MB, and Cascade PN. Cardiovascular MR imaging: technique optimization and detection of disease in clinical practice. *Radiographics*, 2002;22(6):e6.
3. Wang ZJ, Reddy GP, Gotway MB, Yeh BM, and Higgins CB. Cardiovascular shunts: MR imaging evaluation. *Radiographics*, 2003;23 Spec No:S181–194.
4. Choi YH, Park JH, Choe YH, and Yoo SJ. MR imaging of Ebstein's anomaly of the tricuspid valve. *AJR Am J Roentgenol*, 1994;163(3):539–543.
5. Didier D, Saint-Martin C, Lapierre C, et al. Coarctation of the aorta: pre and postoperative evaluation with MRI and MR angiography; correlation with echocardiography and surgery. *Int J Cardiovasc Imaging*, 2006;22(3–4):457–475.
6. Pujadas S, Reddy GP, Weber O, Tan C, Moore P, and Higgins CB. Phase contrast MR imaging to measure changes in collateral blood flow after stenting of recurrent aortic coarctation: initial experience. *J Magn Reson Imaging*, 2006;24(1):72–76.
7. Wald RM and Powell AJ. Simple congenital heart lesions. *J Cardiovasc Magn Reson*, 2006;8(4):619–631.
8. Warnes CA. Transposition of the great arteries. *Circulation*, 2006;114(24):2699–2709.
9. Oosterhof T, Mulder BJ, Vliegen HW, and de Roos A. Cardiovascular magnetic resonance in the follow-up of patients with corrected tetralogy of Fallot: a review. *Am Heart J*, 2006;151(2):265–272.
10. Park JH, Han MC, and Kim CW. MR imaging of congenitally corrected transposition of the great vessels in adults. *AJR Am J Roentgenol*, 1989;153(3):491–494.
11. Dorfman AL and Geva T. Magnetic resonance imaging evaluation of congenital heart disease: conotruncal anomalies. *J Cardiovasc Magn Reson*, 2006;8(4):645–659.
12. Gonzalez-Juanatey C, Testa A, Vidan J, et al. Persistent left superior vena cava draining into the coronary sinus: report of 10 cases and literature review. *Clin Cardiol*, 2004;27(9):515–518.
13. Reddy GP and Higgins CB. Congenital heart disease: measuring physiology with MRI. *Semin Roentgenol*, 1998;33(3):228–238.
14. Weinberg PM and Fogel MA. Cardiac MR imaging in congenital heart disease. *Cardiol Clin*, 1998;16(2):315–348.
15. Hernanz-Schulman M. Vascular rings: a practical approach to imaging diagnosis. *Pediatr Radiol*, 2005;35(10):961–979.
16. Kiaffas MG, Davlouros P, Tsertos F, Andreou J, and Danias PG. Cardiovascular magnetic resonance evaluation of patients with transposition of the great arteries following atrial switch surgical correction. *Hellenic J Cardiol*, 2005;46(1):69–73.

7

Diseases of the Great Vessels

Peter G. Danias, *Cardiovascular MRI: 150 Multiple-Choice Questions and Answers*

1. The study in Fig. 7.1 was acquired in a middle-aged man with chest pain. A transverse T1-weighted spin-echo cardiovascular magnetic resonance imaging (CMR) scan at the level of the bifurcation of the pulmonary artery is presented.

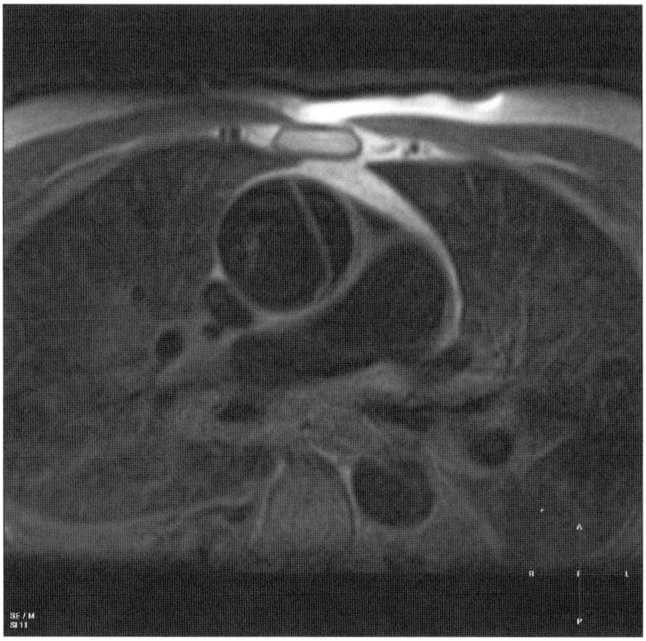

The diagnosis is:

A. Aortic aneurysm with atherosclerosis
B. Aortic coarctation
C. Aortic aneurysm with wall ulcer
D. Aortic aneurysm with dissection
E. Aortic aneurysm with flow artifact

Correct answer is D.

The ascending aorta is dilated and there is a dissection flap clearly visualized in the vessel (Fig. 7.2, *arrows*), establishing the diagnosis of aortic dissection. There is no other sign of other aortic wall pathology, including atherosclerosis or wall ulceration. The aortic arch and isthmus are not visualized in Fig. 7.2, and, thus, the possibility of aortic coarctation cannot be evaluated from this single image. CMR has exquisite sensitivity, specificity, and accuracy for diagnosis of acute thoracic aortic dissection [1–4].

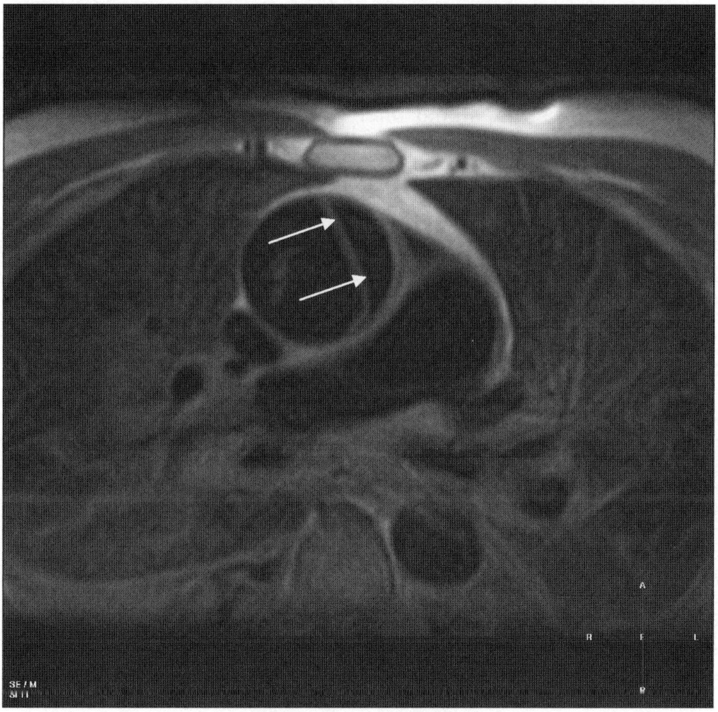

2. In the patient discussed in Question 1, which statement is correct?

A. The larger lumen is the true one and the false lumen (smaller) is thrombosed
B. The larger lumen is the true one and the false lumen (smaller) is not thrombosed
C. The smaller lumen is the true one and the false lumen (larger) is thrombosed
D. The smaller lumen is the true one and the false lumen (larger) is not thrombosed
E. There is no way to tell from the image in Fig. 7.2 which is the true lumen and which is the false lumen

Correct answer is D.

There are imaging findings that can identify the true and false lumens in CMR (and computed tomography [CT] scans). The true lumen is usually smaller and it has edges with the convex side outward (the so called "beak sign") [5]. When there is slow flow or thrombosis, the signal intensity is different inside the true and false lumens. In black blood images, such as the one shown here (Fig. 7.2), a thrombosed lumen would present with intermediate or high signal intensity.

3. The image in Fig. 7.3 is a three-dimensional reconstruction of a contrast-enhanced MR angiography, obtained from a middle-aged man with decreased pulses in the left arm, high sedimentation rate, and fever.

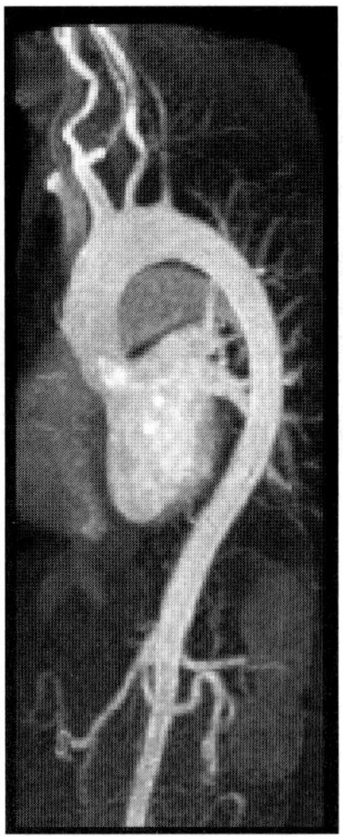

What is a likely diagnosis?

A. Polyarteritis nodosa
B. Takayasu disease
C. Kawasaki disease
D. Aortic dissection
E. Syphilitic aortitis

Correct answer is B.

Takayasu arteritis is an autoimmune vasculitis, characterized by inflammation of the wall of large vessels, typically the aortic arch and the proximal segments of the arch vessels. Takayasu disease is more common in women than in men, and clinically presents with systemic symptoms, signs of inflammation (high sedimentation rate, C-reactive protein, and white cell count), and decreased upper extremity pulses (hence the term "pulseless disease"). Typical imaging findings are wall thickening (best appreciated in T1- or T2-weighted images) with contrast uptake, suggestive of increased blood flow from the vasa vasorum. Luminal stenosis of the large vessels ensues as the wall thickening progresses [6, 7]. The image in Fig. 7.4 demonstrates obliteration of the lumen of the left subclavian artery over a large segment (*arrows*). Polyarteritis nodosa is a vasculitis of medium and small size arteries, frequently affecting the renal arteries. Kawasaki disease affects children and may result in coronary artery aneurysms. Syphilitic aortitis is characterized by ascending aortic aneurysm with vessel wall thickening. There are no signs of dissection in the image presented here (Fig. 7.4).

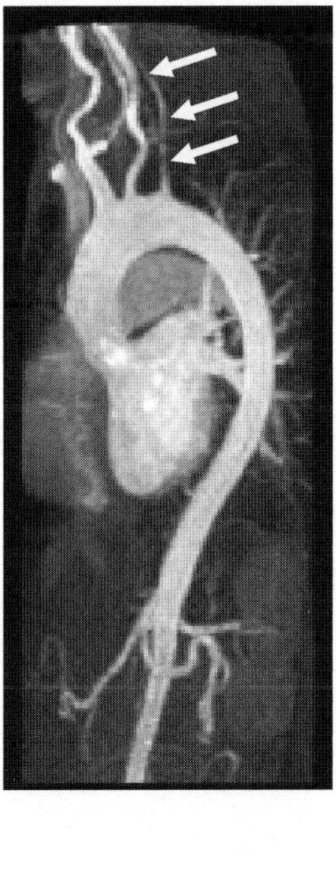

4. An obese patient is referred for CMR for evaluation of cardiomyopathy and shortness of breath. The images in Fig. 7.5 are transverse gradient-echo (white blood) images obtained at the bifurcation of the pulmonary artery *(left panel)* and at the level of the coronary sinus *(right panel).*

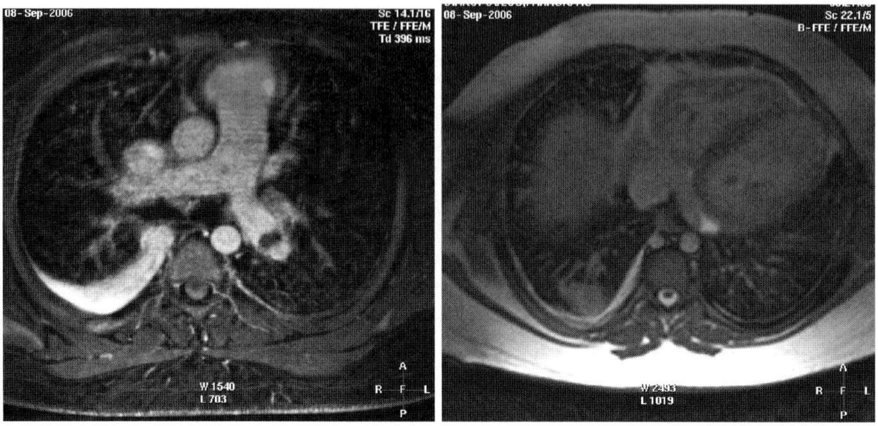

The most likely diagnosis is:

A. Aortic dissection
B. Right lower lobe pneumonia
C. Pulmonary thromboembolic disease
D. Pulmonary hypertension
E. Patent ductus arteriosus

Correct answer is C.

The image on the *left* in Fig. 7.6 demonstrates a low-signal intensity area inside the left pulmonary artery (*black arrow*). There is also a pleural effusion (*Pl.eff*) in the right hemithorax. The image on the *right* in Fig. 7.6 shows a wedge-shaped high-signal area at the right lung base (*white arrow*). These findings are consistent with pulmonary thromboembolic disease with multiple emboli. A right lower lobe pneumonia would explain the findings in the *right panel* image of Fig. 7.6 and the ipsilateral pleural effusion, but not the filling defect inside the left pulmonary artery. There are no signs of aortic dissection or patent ductus arteriosus. No comment can be made regarding the presence of pulmonary hypertension from these images.

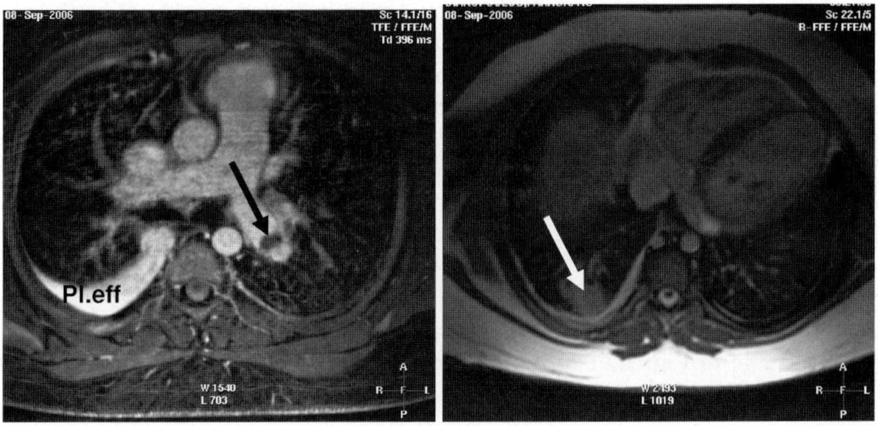

5. Which would be the preferred modality for sequential imaging and follow-up for a 15-year-old patient with Marfan syndrome and mild dilation of the aortic root and the descending thoracic aorta?

A. Contrast-enhanced CT
B. Noncontrast enhanced CT
C. Transesophageal echocardiography (TEE)
D. Transthoracic echocardiography
E. CMR

Correct answer is E.

Contrast-enhanced CT scan, TEE, and MRI are equally accurate for the diagnosis of aortic aneurysms. TEE is a semi-invasive procedure that would not be the preferred modality when serial evaluations are needed and may be more limited for assessment of the aortic arch in certain individuals. Noncontrast CT is adequate to assess aortic dimensions, but the biologic cost from X-ray radiation exposure with serial studies would be considerable for a 15-year-old adolescent. Transthoracic echocardiography may visualize the aortic root well, but usually cannot adequately evaluate the descending thoracic aorta. CMR can provide accurate dimensions of the entire aorta, can assess for possible aortic valve insufficiency and has no adverse biologic effects. Therefore, MRI would be the preferred modality for sequential follow-up in this adolescent with Marfan syndrome [8, 9].

6. The image in Fig. 7.7 is obtained from a three-dimensional reconstruction of the aorta in a patient undergoing contrast-enhanced CMR.

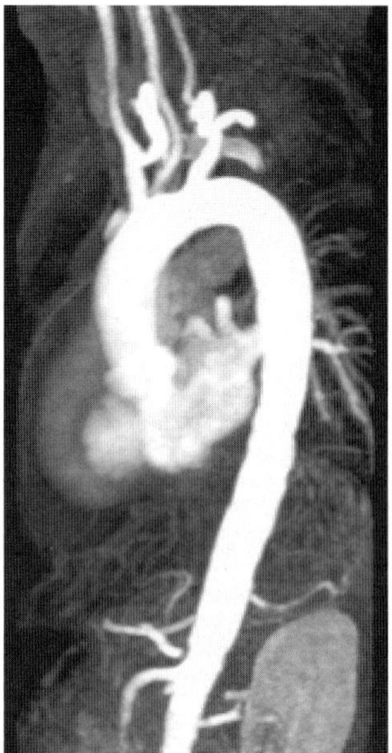

Which of the following statements best describes the pertinent findings in this image?

A. Aortic coarctation
B. Aneurysmal dilation of the sinuses of Valsalva
C. Atherosclerosis of the descending aorta including a significant ostial stenosis of the celiac artery
D. Atherosclerosis of the descending aorta including a significant ostial stenosis of the superior mesenteric artery
E. Aortic dissection

Correct answer is C.

In the image in Fig. 7.8, the superior mesenteric artery (*SMA*) and celiac artery are indicated. The *arrows* demonstrate an irregular contour of the descending thoracic aorta, suggestive of atherosclerosis. At the ostium of the celiac artery, a signal void is present, suggestive of a significant stenosis. The origin of the SMA has no significant stenosis. There is no evidence of coarctation or aortic dissection. The aorta at the level of the sinuses of Valsalva has a normal diameter. Contrast-enhanced CMR angiography of the thoracic and abdominal vessels can readily demonstrate pathology in these territories [10, 11].

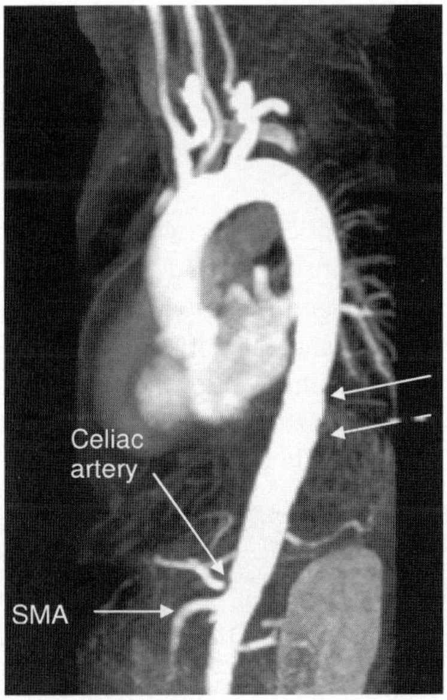

7. **The study in Fig. 7.9 was acquired in a 65-year-old patient. The left panel is a single slice from the gadolinium-enhanced CMR angiogram. The right panel is a transverse slice at the site of the aortic pathology.**

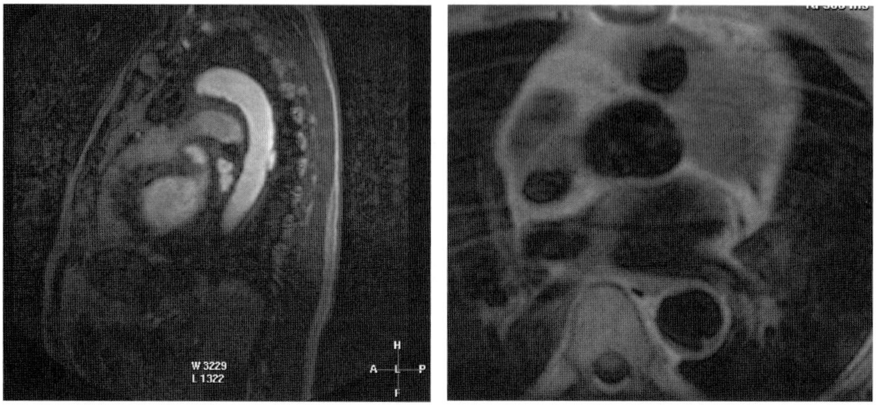

The diagnosis is:

A. Aortic aneurysm
B. Aortic coarctation
C. Aortic ulcer
D. Aortic dissection
E. Williams syndrome

Correct answer is C.

Aortic ulcers involve atherosclerotic aortic walls, carry the same significance as aortic dissection and can be readily diagnosed with CMR [12, 13]. The aortic wall ulceration seen at the CMR angiogram on the left (arrow) may be misinterpreted as dissection with presence of true and false lumens, but the transverse black-blood slice (dashed arrow, right panel) demonstrates that there is an atherosclerotic plaque with intra-plaque ulceration. There is no evidence for aortic aneurysm, coarctation, or supravalvular aortic stenosis (Williams syndrome).

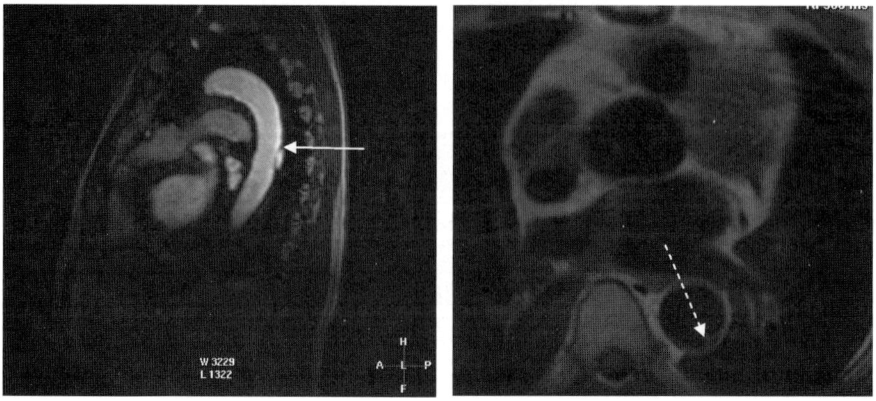

8. Figure 7.10 shows a T1-weighted transverse spin-echo CMR image that was obtained in an asymptomatic 65-year-old man, who was referred for evaluation of ascending aortic dilation.

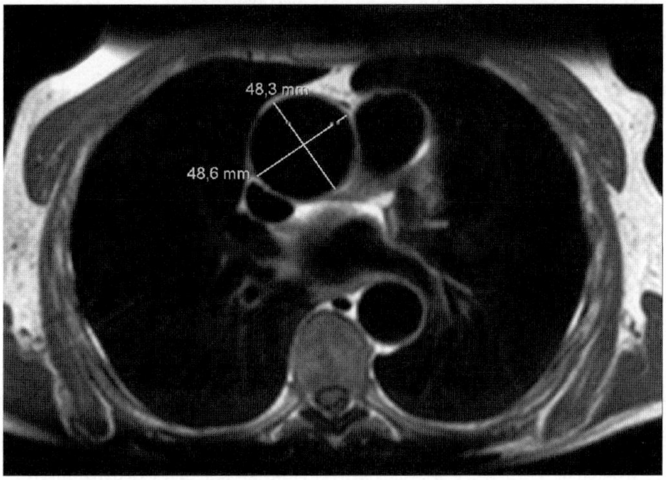

What is the most appropriate next step?

A. Referral to a cardiothoracic surgeon for immediate surgical therapy
B. Reassurance; no further testing required, as long as the patient remains asymptomatic
C. Referral for CT angiography to best delineate the aortic anatomy
D. Cardiac catheterization and coronary angiography
E. Follow-up CMR examination in a few months

Correct answer is E.

The image demonstrates dilation of the ascending aorta without evidence of aortic dissection. The cumulative risk of rupture of a thoracic aortic aneurysm is related to its diameter. In a large analysis of 1,600 patients, aortic size was a very strong predictor of rupture, dissection, and mortality. In patients with an aorta with maximal diameter of 6 cm, the annual risk is high: rupture (3.6%), dissection (3.7%), death (10.8%), and rupture, dissection, or death (14.1%) [14]. The risk is higher in patients with Marfan syndrome or other connective tissue synthesis disorders, those with bicuspid aortic valves, and those with a strong family history of aortic rupture. In the case presented here, the aortic diameter case is less than 50 mm and the annual risk of rupture in patients who are not high risk with this aortic size is on the order of 4%, justifying a watchful approach. Follow-up testing is indicated to assess the rate of expansion. CT scanning does not add any more information to the CMR examination, and diagnostic cardiac catheterization is not indicated at this time.

9. Which of the following statements best describes the clinical usefulness of CMR for diagnosis of acute thoracic aortic dissection?

A. The diagnosis relies on the three-dimensional reconstruction of the aorta obtained from contrast-enhanced MR angiography
B. A positive finding should always be confirmed with a contrast-enhanced CT scan before surgery is undertaken
C. CMR, contrast-enhanced CT scan, and TEE have comparable accuracy for making the diagnosis of aortic dissection
D. The diagnostic value of CMR is roughly equal to that of transthoracic echocardiography
E. CMR is useful in identifying the dissection flap, but has little, if any, value for assessment of complications of acute thoracic aortic dissection

Correct answer is C.

The sensitivity and specificity of CMR, CT scan, and TEE are all very high (well above 95%), and all three tests are considered to be equally good in establishing the diagnosis of acute aortic dissection [1, 2, 4, 15]. Transthoracic echocardiography is significantly inferior and may be of some value for ascending aorta dissections. Similar to CT scanning, diagnosis with CMR is typically made from the source images, and certainly does not *rely on* the three-dimensional reconstructions. Besides identifying the dissection flap, CMR has also value in assessing complications of aortic dissection, such as hemopericardium and aortic valvular insufficiency.

10. Figure 7.11 is a black blood transverse image at the level of the aortic arch.

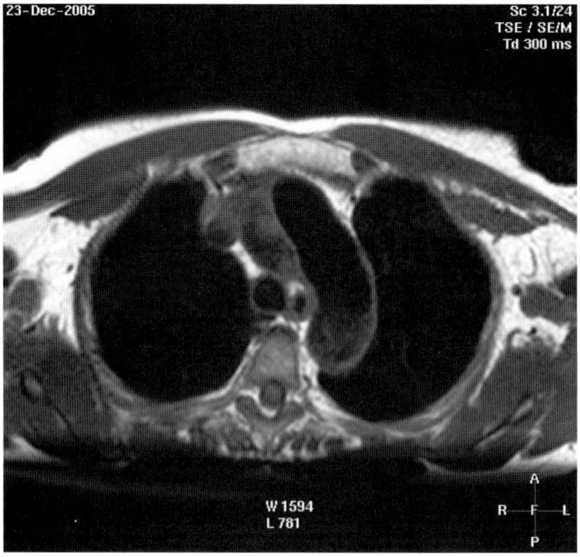

What is the likely diagnosis?

A. Coarctation
B. Persistent left superior vena cava
C. Aortic ring
D. Aortic dissection
E. Aortic wall ulcer

Correct answer is D.

In Fig. 7.12, the dissection flap is labeled with *arrows*. Although this is not always the case, in this patient, the flow inside the false lumen (*FL*) is slower, accounting for the intermediate signal inside the false lumen (incomplete suppression of the blood pool signal), compared with the true lumen (*TL*). The superior vena cava (*SVC*) is at the expected location, and there is no persistent left superior vena cava. The trachea (*T*) is also indicated.

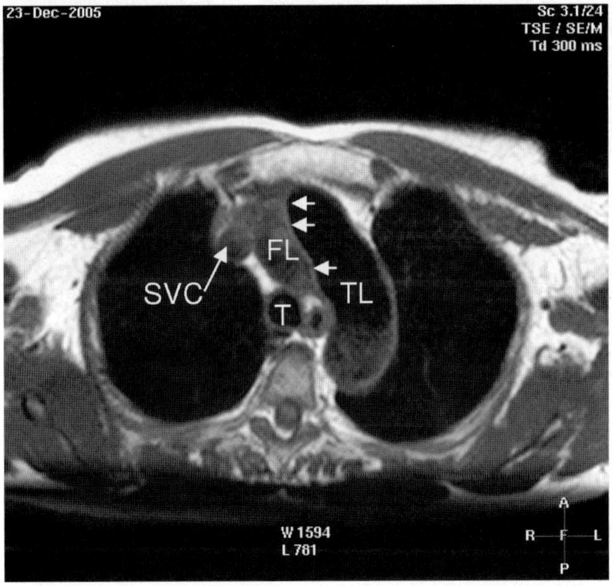

11. Several years after an automobile accident, a middle-aged man is noted to have an abnormal chest X-ray and is referred for a CMR study. The image in Fig. 7.13 is a maximal intensity projection (MIP) of the aorta, obtained from three-dimensional contrast-enhanced CMR angiography.

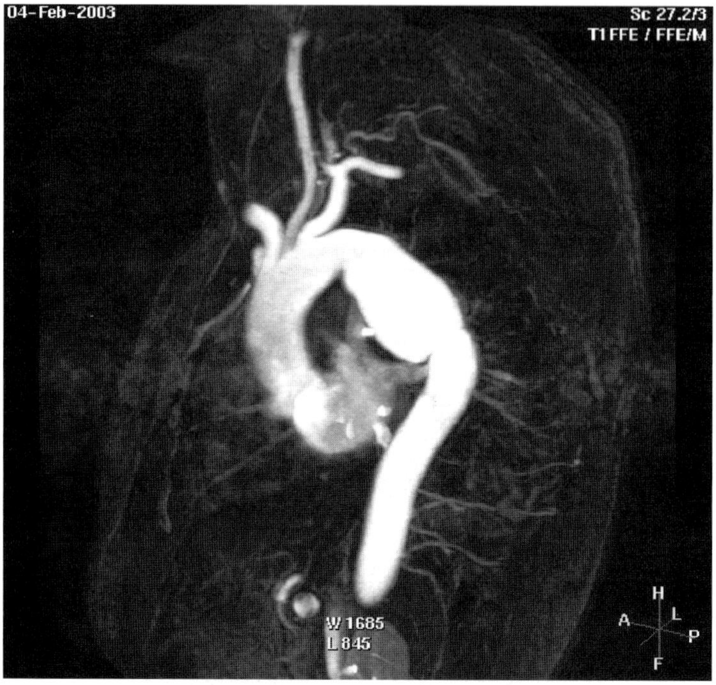

What is the most likely diagnosis?

A. Aortic coarctation
B. Interrupted aortic arch
C. Aortic rupture
D. Aortic pseudoaneurysm
E. Takayasu arteritis

Correct answer is D.

Aortic pseudoaneurysms are commonly post-traumatic, tend to occur at the proximal part of the descending thoracic aorta after deceleration accidents, and may go undiagnosed until later [16]. Partial aortic rupture may be initially walled of by a thrombus and later become calcified. Indeed, this patient had heavy calcification of the aorta at the site of the pseudoaneurysm. Coarctation usually has poststenotic dilation of the descending thoracic aorta, but, in this case, there is no focal stenosis of the aortic lumen. Takayasu arteritis usually involves the arch and may result in aneurysm formation. Takayasu disease is more common in women, and, given the clinical scenario, it would be a very unlikely cause for the aortic pathology in this patient.

12. The images in Fig. 7.14 are transverse T1-weighted spin-echo CMR images at the inferior cardiac border, before *(A)* and after *(B)* contrast administration (0.1 mmol/kg gadolinium).

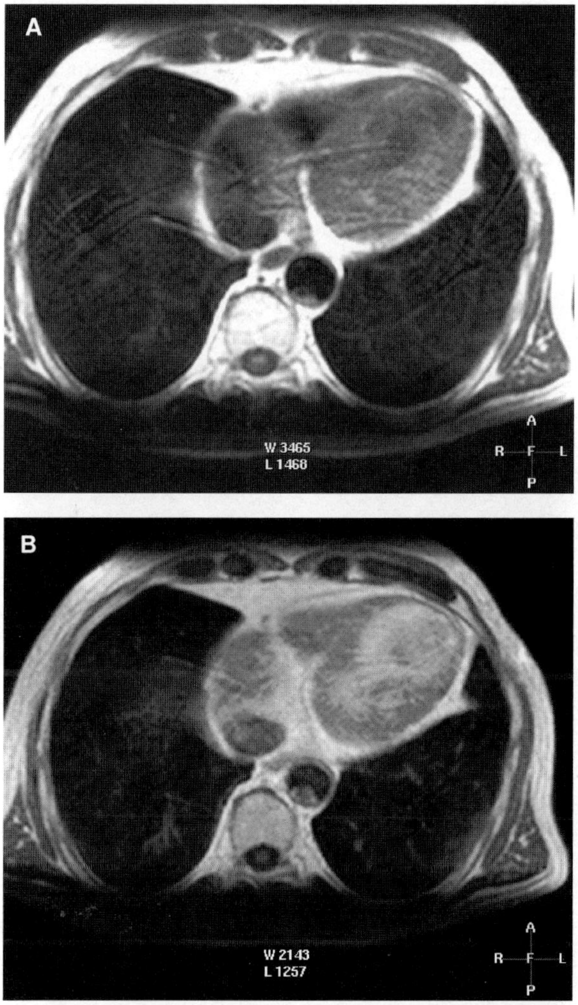

What statement best describes the findings from these images?

A. There is significant coronary and aortic atherosclerotic disease
B. There is dissection of the descending thoracic aorta
C. There is dilation of the coronary sinus
D. There is evidence of myocardial infarction in the distribution of the left circumflex coronary artery
E. There are no abnormal findings in this image

Correct answer is A.

There are two pertinent findings in these images. First, there is significant wall thinning at the distal intraventricular septum and apex. This is evident in both the precontrast and postcontrast scans, although, in the noncontrast-enhanced image (Fig. 7.15A, *black arrows*), the slow flow in the area of the previous infarction does not allow for complete blood pool signal suppression inside the left ventricle. After contrast administration, the slow flow creates a brighter rim that better delineates the thinned out myocardium (Fig. 7.15B, *black arrows*). The second significant finding is a large atheromatous plaque in the descending thoracic aorta (Fig. 7.15A, *white arrows*). The plaque takes up contrast predominantly in its outer layer, where there is more neovascularization (Fig. 7.15B, *white arrows*). The central low-signal area represents the lipid core and does not enhance after contrast administration.

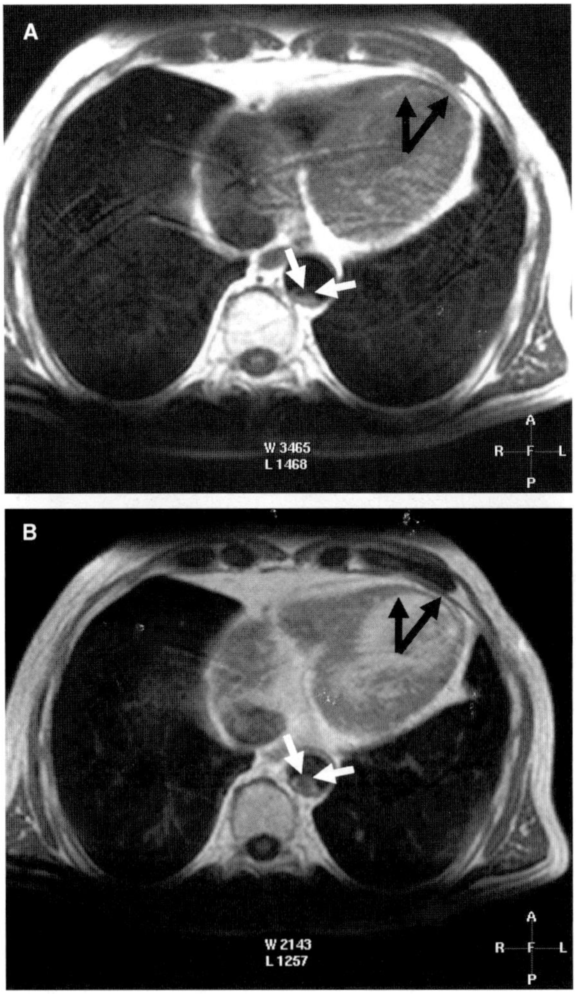

13. The image in Fig. 7.16 is a single frame from a cine CMR study at the base of the heart in a middle-aged patient with chest pain.

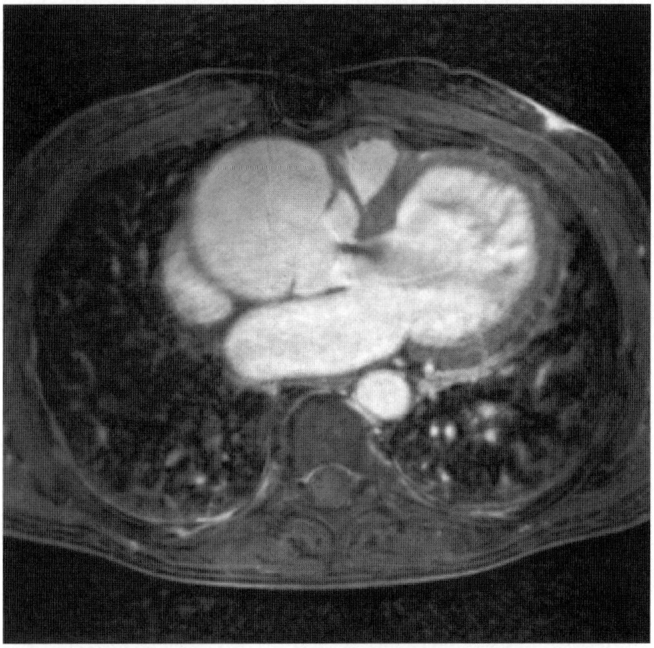

Based on the findings of this image, all of the following should be considered *except* for:

A. Aortic dissection of the ascending thoracic aorta
B. Aortic aneurysm
C. Aortic valve regurgitation
D. Previous sternotomy
E. Severe chronic mitral regurgitation

Correct answer is E.

The image in Fig. 7.17 demonstrates aortic root dilation with a proximal dissection flap (*black arrows*), establishing the diagnosis of ascending aortic dissecting aneurysm. There is also a signal void in the left ventricular outflow tract, suggesting that the image represents ventricular diastole, and that aortic regurgitation is present. During diastole, one would not expect to see a signal void associated with mitral regurgitation, and the size of the left atrium argues against chronic severe mitral insufficiency. The *white arrowhead* demonstrates artifact from sternal wires from a previous thoracotomy.

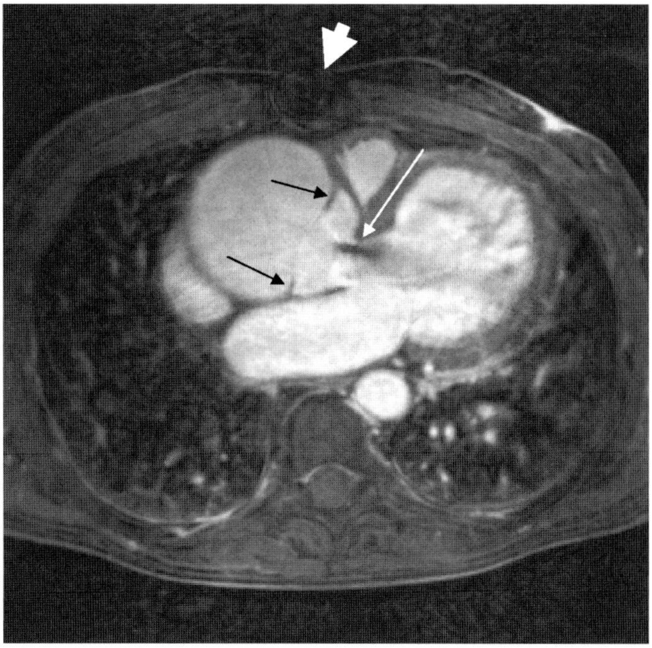

References

1. Moore AG, Eagle KA, Bruckman D, et al. Choice of computed tomography, transesophageal echocardiography, magnetic resonance imaging, and aortography in acute aortic dissection: International Registry of Acute Aortic Dissection (IRAD). Am J Cardiol, 2002; 89(10):1235–1238.
2. Nienaber CA, von Kodolitsch Y, Nicolas V, et al. The diagnosis of thoracic aortic dissection by noninvasive imaging procedures. N Engl J Med, 1993;328(1):1–9.
3. Shiga T, Wajima Z, Apfel CC, Inoue T, and Ohe Y. Diagnostic accuracy of transesophageal echocardiography, helical computed tomography, and magnetic resonance imaging for suspected thoracic aortic dissection: systematic review and meta-analysis. Arch Intern Med, 2006;166(13):1350–1356.
4. Sommer T, Fehske W, Holzknecht N, et al. Aortic dissection: a comparative study of diagnosis with spiral CT, multiplanar transesophageal echocardiography, and MR imaging. Radiology, 1996;199(2):347–352.
5. LePage MA, Quint LE, Sonnad SS, Deeb GM, and Williams DM. Aortic dissection: CT features that distinguish true lumen from false lumen. AJR Am J Roentgenol, 2001; 177(1):207–211.
6. Meller J, Grabbe E, Becker W, and Vosshenrich R. Value of F-18 FDG hybrid camera PET and MRI in early Takayasu aortitis. Eur Radiol, 2003;13(2):400–405.
7. Yamada I, Numano F, and Suzuki S. Takayasu arteritis: evaluation with MR imaging. Radiology, 1993;188(1):89–94.
8. Givehchian M, Kramer U, Miller S, et al. Aortic root remodeling: functional MRI as an accurate tool for complete follow-up. Thorac Cardiovasc Surg, 2005;53(5):267–273.
9. Meijboom LJ, Groenink M, van der Wall EE, Romkes H, Stoker J, and Mulder BJ. Aortic root asymmetry in Marfan patients; evaluation by magnetic resonance imaging and comparison with standard echocardiography. Int J Card Imaging, 2000;16(3):161–168.
10. Leiner T. Magnetic resonance angiography of abdominal and lower extremity vasculature. Top Magn Reson Imaging, 2005;16(1):21–66.
11. Nael K, Laub G, and Finn JP. Three-dimensional contrast-enhanced MR angiography of the thoraco-abdominal vessels. Magn Reson Imaging Clin N Am, 2005;13(2):359–380.
12. Hayashi H, Matsuoka Y, Sakamoto I, et al. Penetrating atherosclerotic ulcer of the aorta: imaging features and disease concept. Radiographics, 2000;20(4):995–1005.
13. Mohiaddin RH, McCrohon J, Francis JM, Barbir M, and Pennell DJ. Contrast-enhanced magnetic resonance angiogram of penetrating aortic ulcer. Circulation, 2001;103(4):E18–19.
14. Elefteriades JA. Natural history of thoracic aortic aneurysms: indications for surgery, and surgical versus nonsurgical risks. Ann Thorac Surg, 2002;74(5):S1877–1880; discussion S1892–1878.
15. Hartnell GG. Imaging of aortic aneurysms and dissection: CT and MRI. *J Thorac Imaging*, 2001;16(1):35–46.
16. Gurkan S, Sunar H, Canbaz S, and Duran E. Late manifestation of a pseudoaneurysm in the descending thoracic aorta. *Vasa*, 2006;35(2):112–114.

Index